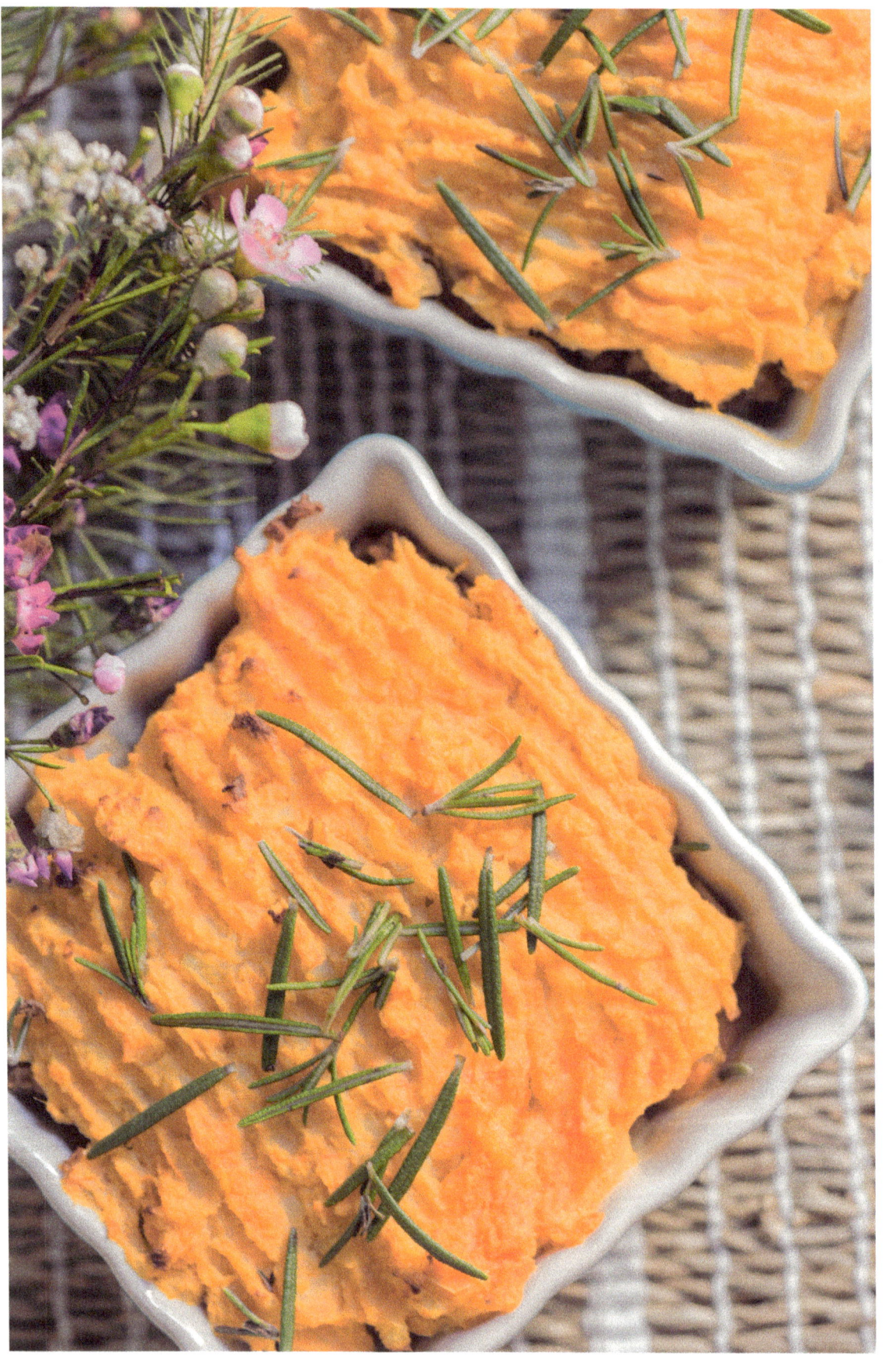

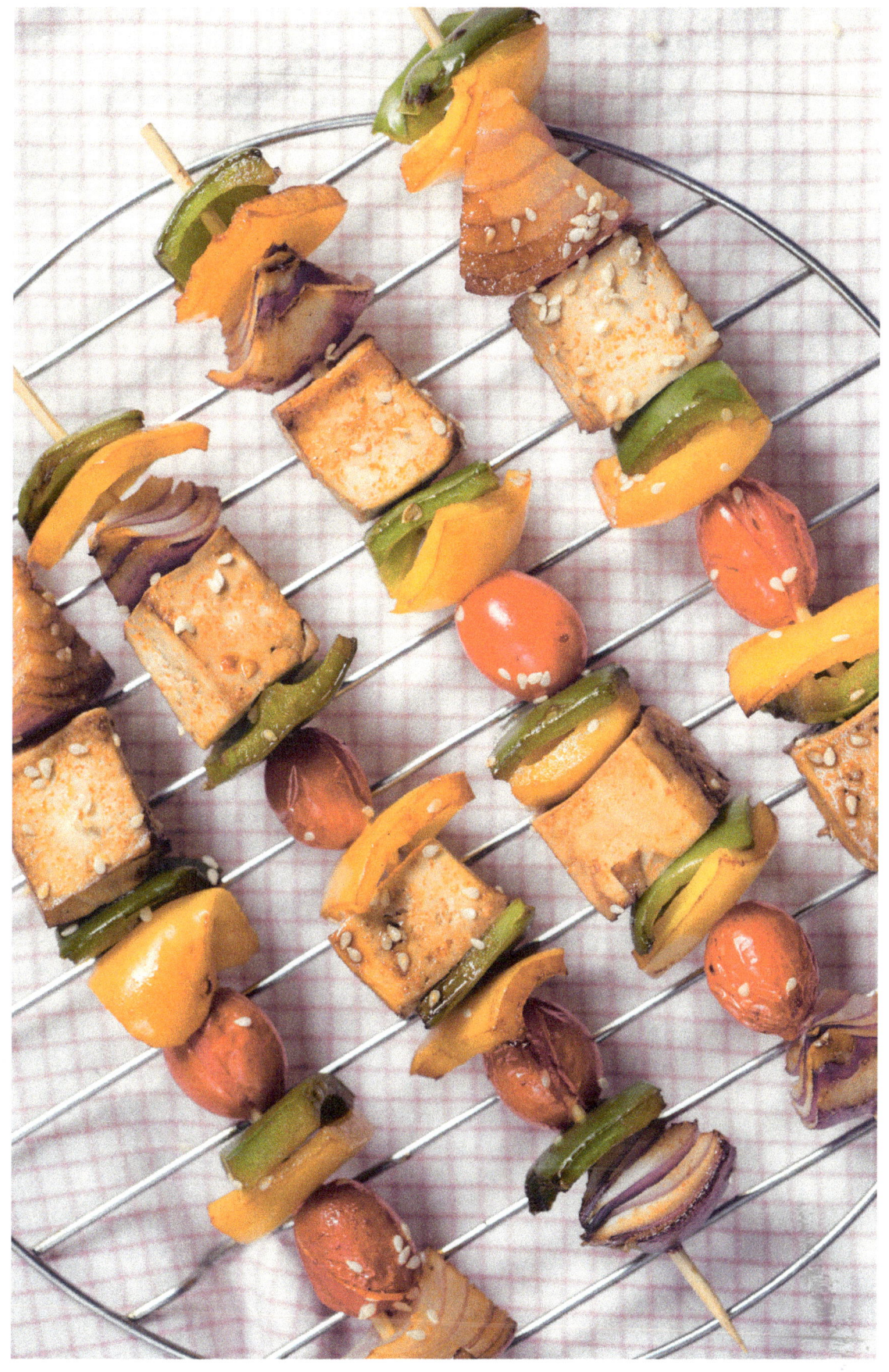

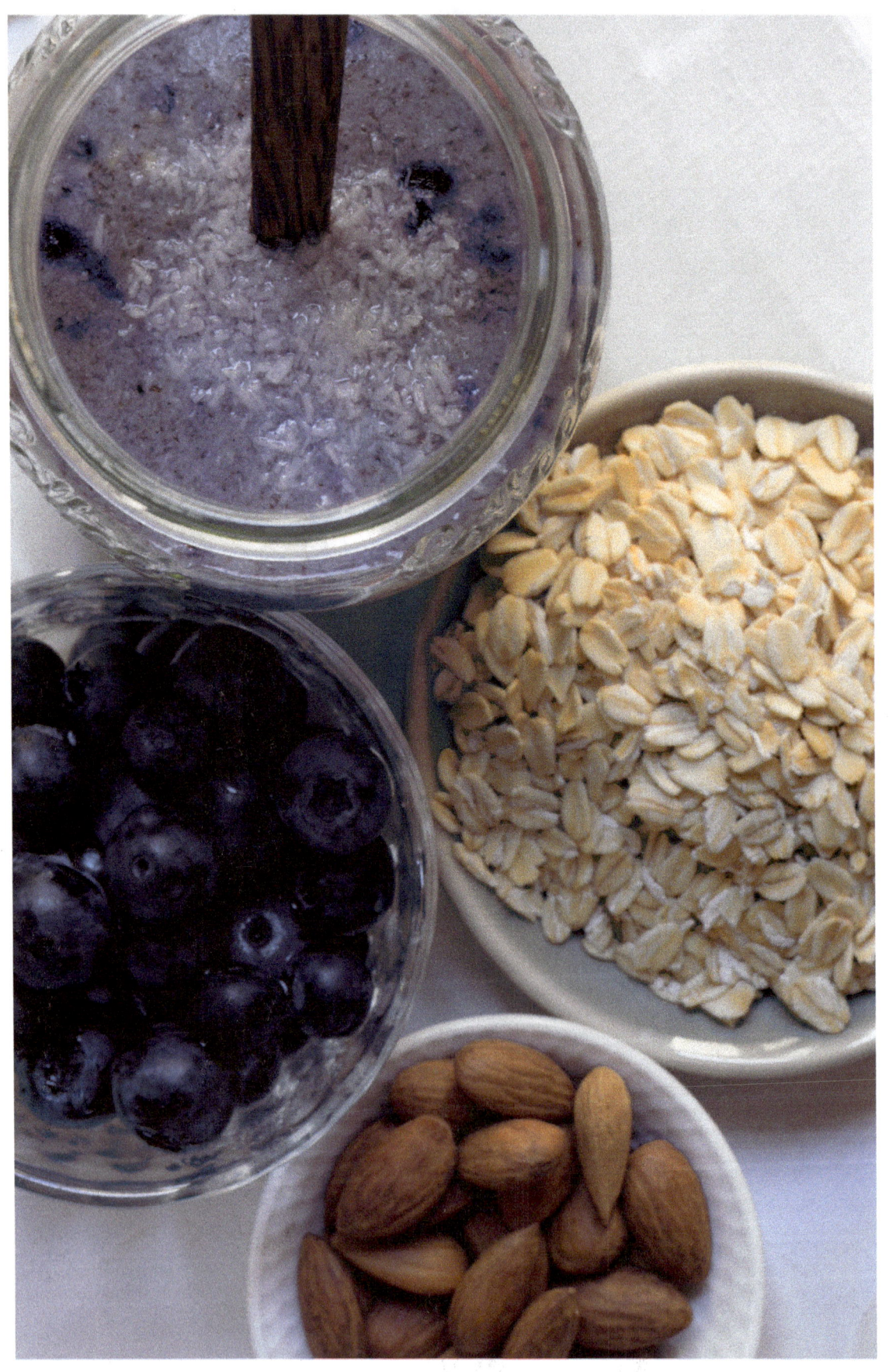

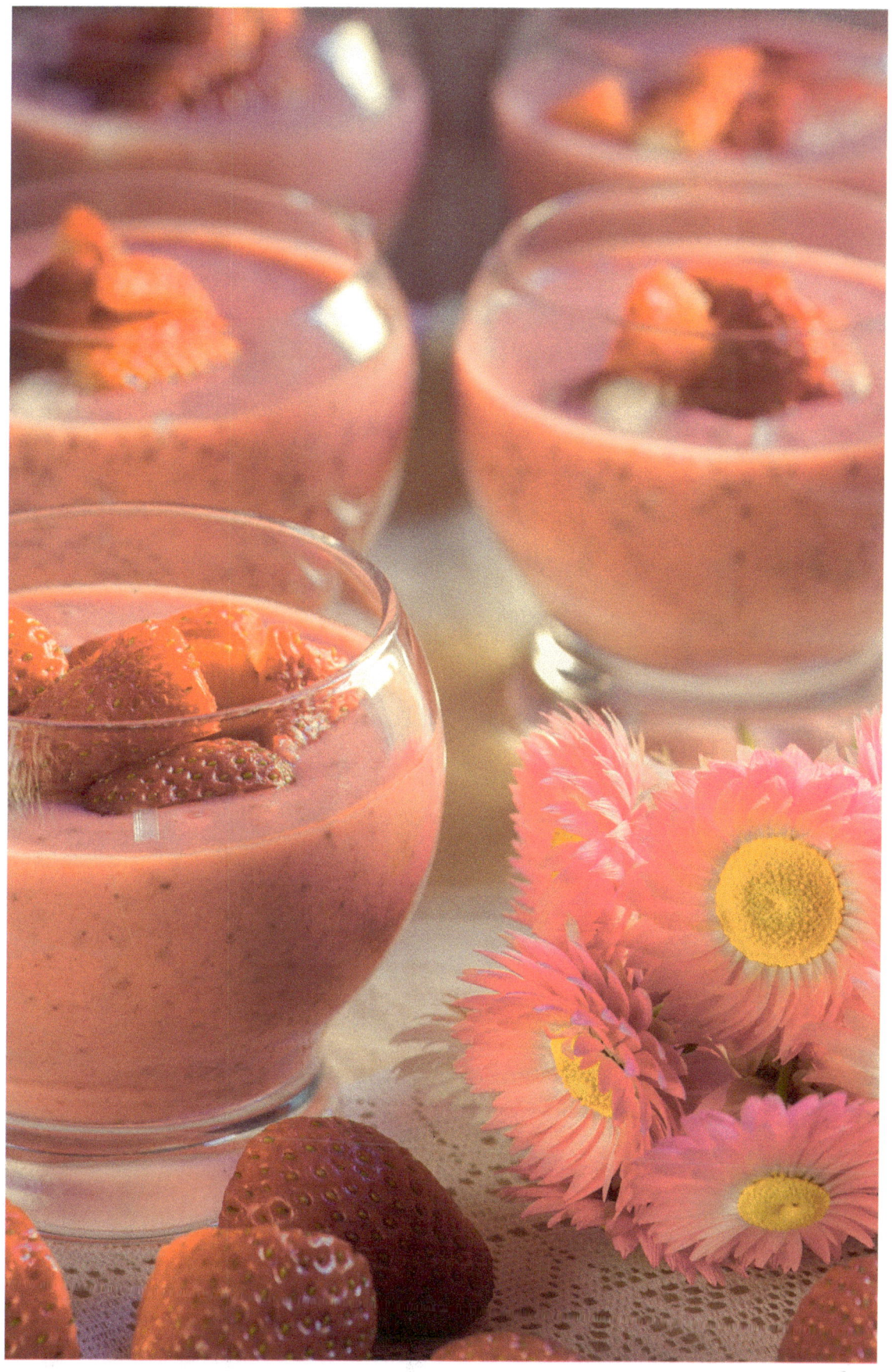

65+ high-protein plant-based recipes to inspire you.

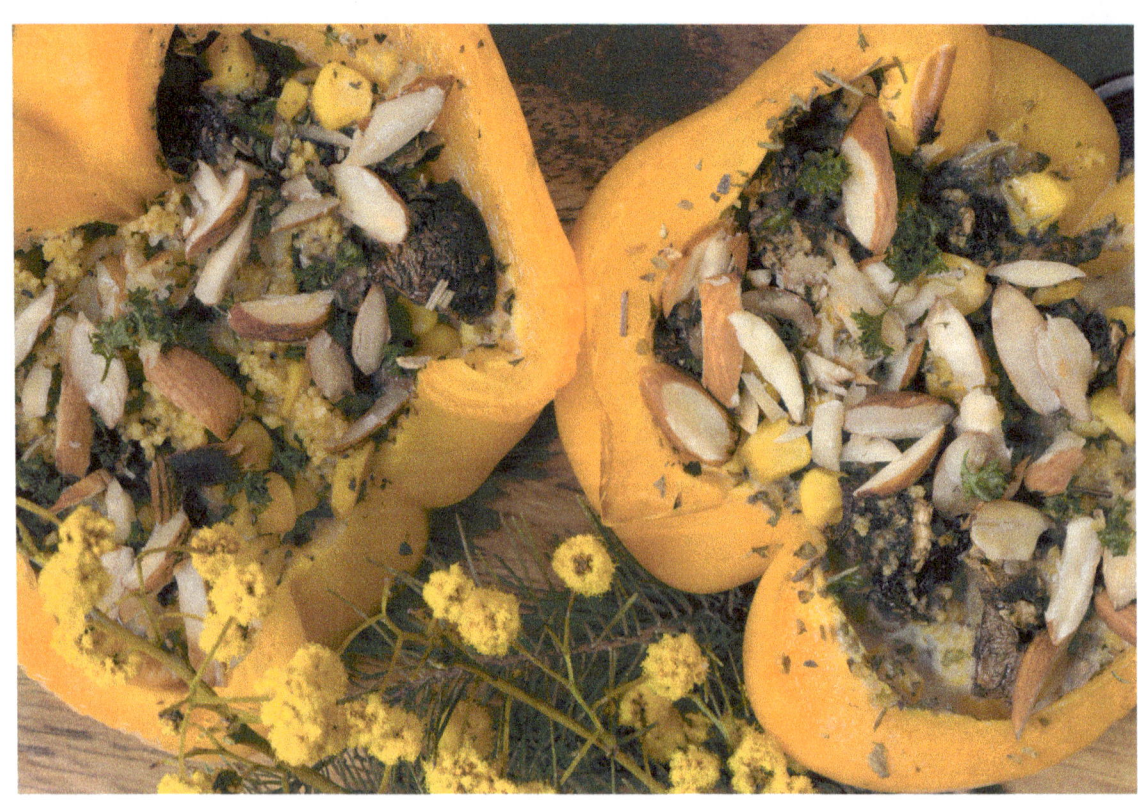

The high-protein PLANT-BASED COOKBOOK

Vegan-friendly.

Planet-friendly.

ANISE & GREEN

This book aims to inspire healthy eating choices through high-protein plant-based meals. These recipes are planet friendly, because vegan-friendly plant-based foods require fewer environmental resources than meat or dairy, and are therefore kinder to our planet.

Comments and suggestions for future editions are warmly received at *www.aniseandgreen.com*.

Ingredients and nutritional information

Any of the speciality ingredients used in this book should be available from good health-food stores. Nutritional information is provided on a best-effort basis and the exact nutritional values will vary according to the brands of ingredients used. Whilst this book does not endorse specific brands, for listings please contact Anise & Green. The information in this book is not intended to replace or be a substitute for health and nutrition advice from your healthcare provider.

ISBN 978-0-6450542-1-7

Published in 2021 © Anise and Green.

All rights reserved. No part of this publication may be reproduced, stored in a retrieval system, or transmitted in any way or by any means, electronic, mechanical, photocopying, recording or otherwise without the prior written permission of the copyright holder.

The moral rights of the author have been asserted.

Recipes, photography and design: Jennifer Delmarre.

Editor: Bridget Blair.

Set in *"Rosarivo"*, *"Eufoniem One, Locomotype"* and *"Reforma, PampaType / Universidad Nacional de Córdoba [AR]"*.

Ethical-trading policy

At Anise & Green, we believe in reaching for an ethical and sustainable way of life – with respect for the environment and proper regard of the resources we use. Books are printed in very short runs or only when an order has been received. This model of book manufacturing reduces waste and greenhouse emissions and conserves valuable natural resources.

DEDICATION

To Toppy, Marta, Tickle, Buffy and Enzo for your happiness and joy.

ANISE & GREEN: THE HIGH-PROTEIN PLANT-BASED COOKBOOK

CONTENTS

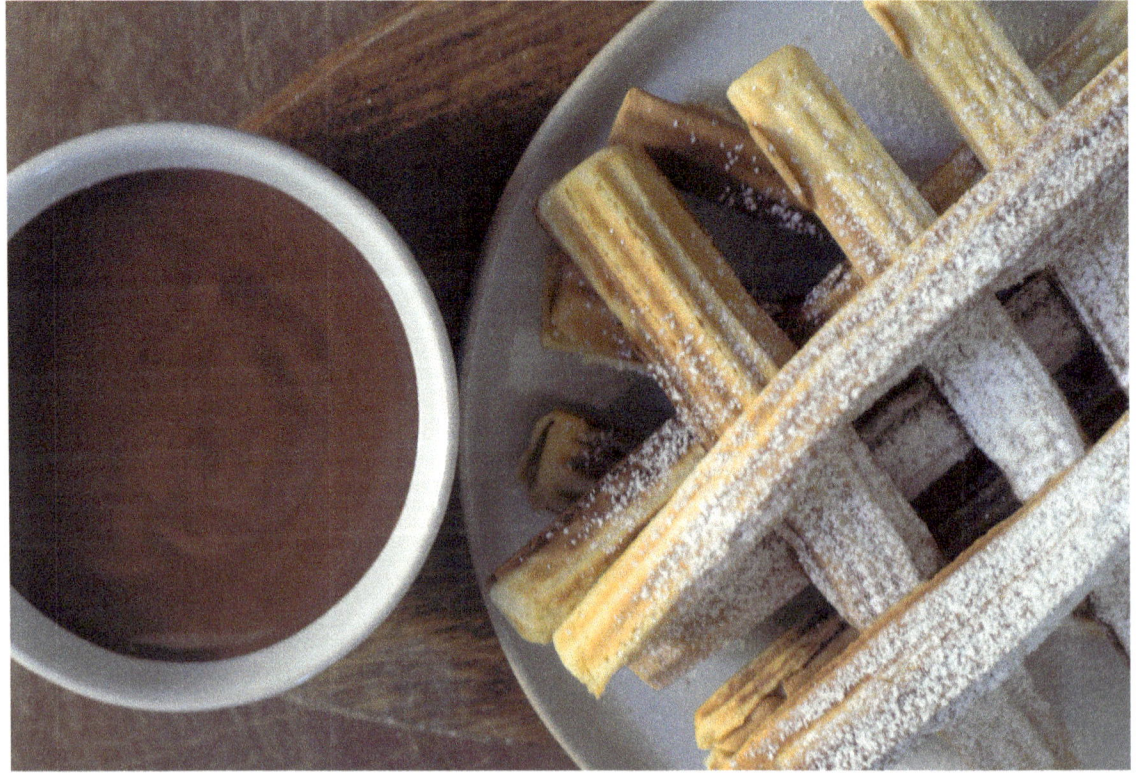

1	Introduction
7	Pantry list
17	Soups
31	Snacks & dips
55	Mains
105	Marinades
113	Salads
125	Dressings
135	Desserts
149	Drinks
160	Resources
165	Index

ANISE & GREEN: THE HIGH-PROTEIN PLANT-BASED COOKBOOK

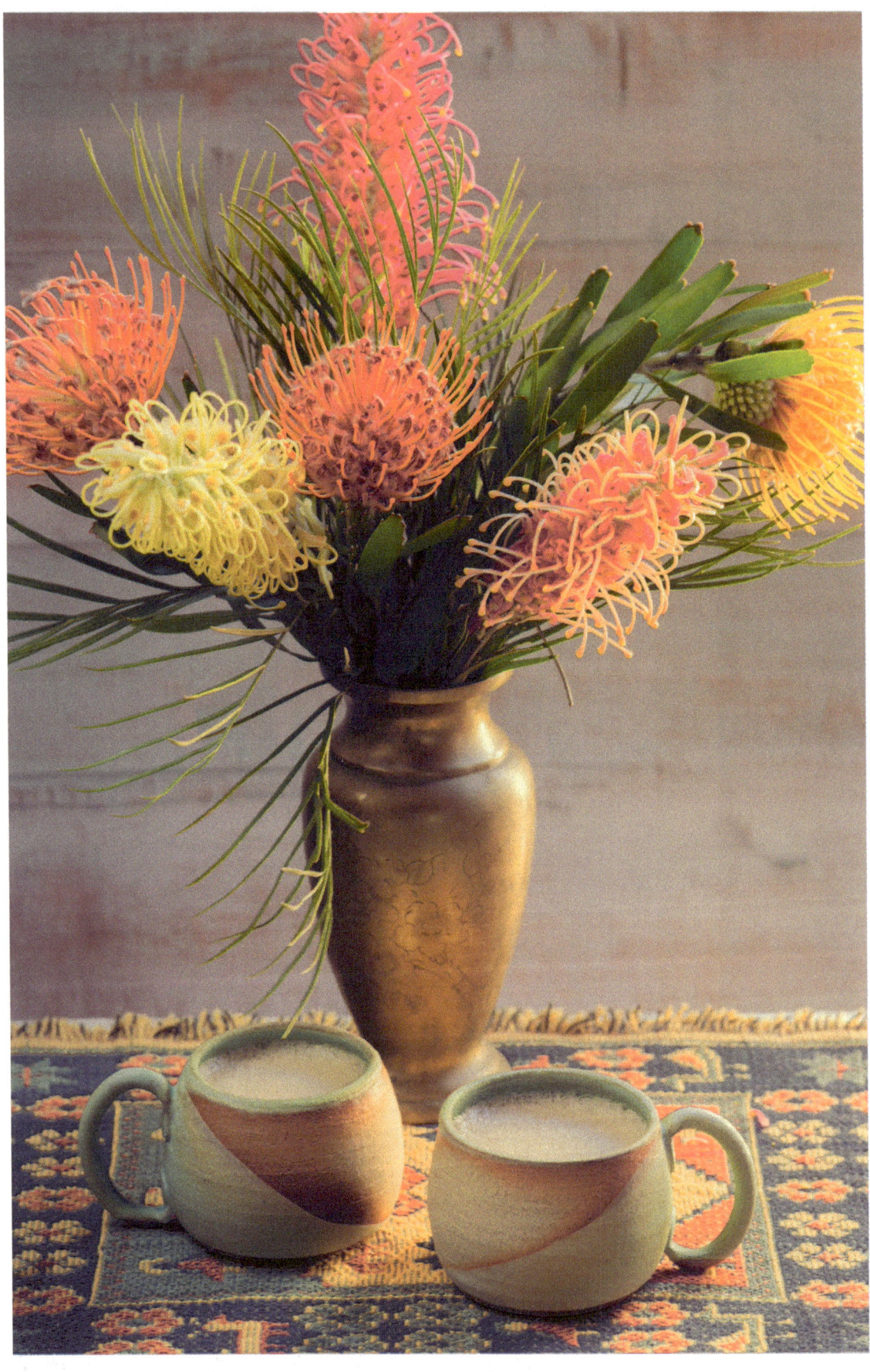

INTRODUCTION

Would you like to eat both high-protein and plant-based food but think it is not possible? We have good news for you – not only is it possible but it's easy and fun, and this book shows you how! Packed full of ideas for starters, snacks mains, salads, drinks and desserts, it contains a range of possibilities to try out, adapt and make your own.

Many high-protein foods are high fat and therefore also high-calorie foods. This book helps to redress that. With these recipes, you can quickly and easily increase the proportion of protein in your meals whilst keeping calories under control. This is particularly important if you plan to start a new exercise or calorie-controlled programme, and you need to reduce your overall calorie intake whilst safeguarding your protein intake. All recipes are vegan-friendly too!

Protein is a macronutrient responsible for playing many critical roles in the body. It is important for your skin, hair and organs and supports enzyme, hormone and antibody production in the body. Protein supports muscle development and regeneration, which in turn helps raise your metabolic rate and favours weight loss. Additionally, eating meals containing a high proportion of protein helps you to feel fuller for longer – making it easier to reduce the amount of food you eat.[1]

There is no 'one size fits all' figure to determine the amount of energy and therefore calories a person requires – this should be determined by your nutritionist, healthcare provider or dietician. However, counting calories is a useful method for

> *Many high-protein foods are high fat and therefore also high-calorie foods. This book helps to redress that.*

---

1   K Gunnars, *Protein intake – how much protein should you eat per day?*, Healthline website, accessed November 2020. https://www.healthline.com/nutrition/how-much-protein-per-day

measuring and tracking overall energy intake and is important for those seeking to lose or gain weight. Calories in food are quoted in 'kcal', although some systems use metric kilojoules ('kJ'). Many online calculators allow you to convert between the two units. **The recipes in this book all contain fewer than 400 calories per serving.**

Protein, fat and carbohydrates are called 'macronutrients' and they determine, among other things, the energy you gain from your food each day. Our bodies burn more calories from 1 gram of fat (9 calories) than they do from 1 gram of protein (4 calories). Therefore if your recipe contained 10g of fat and 10g of protein, your body would generate more energy from fat than protein from that meal. Officially, a food is considered 'high protein' if 20% or more of its calorie content is generated from protein.[2] **All of the recipes in this book provide at least 20% of the total energy from protein.**

Determining the proportion of calories provided by each macronutrient (protein, fat and carbohydrates) in a food or a meal is often called 'counting macros'. This method makes it easy for you to track and increase the relative proportion of calories provided by protein that you consume. **The counting macros method is the approach we have used to develop recipes in this book.**

The general recommended daily intake (RDI) of protein in grams is 0.8 times your weight in kilograms. This is the minimum level of protein you should aim to consume per day.[3] For example, a person weighing 65kg should consume at least 52g of protein per day. This figure varies according to gender and age and, to some extent, activity level.

Proteins are comprised of chains of amino acids. These chains determine the 'amino acid profile' of the food. A 'complete' protein has all of the amino acids in its profile. An example of a complete vegan protein is soy. Soy also provides omega-3s and other nutrients and is low in fat and carbohydrates; it is therefore particularly good for slimming and weight loss.

Some proteins are 'incomplete' because they do not contain all the amino acids required for a full amino acid profile. By combining complementary protein sources, for example, a

All of the recipes in this book provide at least 20% of the total energy from protein.

---

2 European Commission, *Nutrition claims*, EC website, accessed November 2020. https://ec.europa.eu/food/safety/labelling_nutrition/claims/nutrition_claims_en

3 Australian National Health and Medical Research Council, *Protein*, Nutrient Reference Values for Australia and New Zealand (NRV)website, accessed November 2020. https://www.nrv.gov.au/nutrients/protein

grain (e.g. rice) and a legume (e.g. beans), we ensure our meals have complete amino acid profiles. **All of the recipes in this book provide complete amino acid profiles.**

Seitan is a protein derived from wheat gluten and is fairly easy to make at home. Depending on where you live it may be possible to source raw seitan from health food stores. You can use raw seitan in place of tofu in many recipes in this book, such as *'Tantalising tortillas'* on page 56 and *'Sweet potato, ginger and barley soup'* on page 26.

Typically, when we eat food containing a relatively high proportion of carbohydrates, our overall calorie intake is high. This is because carbohydrates are high in energy and, depending on what type we eat and what we eat them with, we can eat a lot of carbohydrates before we feel full.

Carbohydrates provide energy to our bodies and do not provide additional nutrition.[4] This is one reason why limiting the quantity of carbohydrates that you eat in a day can be a safe way to reduce your overall calorie intake. A great way to start is to minimise or eliminate the use of added sugar, a carbohydrate that causes weight gain.[5] **The recipes in this book contain less than 50g carbohydrates per serving.**

Healthy fats are important to include in a plant-based diet. Our bodies require small quantities of healthy fats to absorb fat-soluble vitamins, including vitamins A, D, E and K. The trick is to choose healthy fats and avoid processed foods that likely contain poorer-quality fats. Our recommendation is to choose extra-virgin olive oil (see page 12), coconut or avocado oil for cooking, as these have high smoke points. These can be supplemented with small quantities of hemp-seed and flax-seed oils that contain highly beneficial fats with omega-3 fatty acids. Hemp and flax-seed oils are delicious in cold dishes and are ***not*** recommended for cooking on high heat as they do not have high smoke points.

Lots of fresh fruit and veggies are great choices for salads or side dishes. Not only do they provide an abundance of micronutrients like vitamins but they also contain lots of fibre. Fibre helps us to feel full and improves digestion. Likewise, whole grains contain more fibre and are better choices than

The recipes in this book contain fewer than 50g carbohydrates per serving.

---

4   Australian National Health and Medical Research Council, *Carbohydrate*, NRV website, accessed November 2020. https://www.nrv.gov.au/nutrients/carbohydrate

5   LiveLighter, *Tips for reducing sugar intake*, Live Lighter website, accessed November 2020. https://livelighter.com.au/Top-Tips/Cut-Back-on-Sugar

processed white grains. For example, choose brown or red rice instead of white rice, wholemeal bread instead of white, or wholemeal pasta in place of regular pasta.[6]

Lifestyle is important – a healthy level of activity is arguably as important as diet. Exercise burns calories, therefore it makes sense that a healthy weight is best maintained by a nutritious, calorie-controlled diet in combination with exercise. As our bodies burn calories with exercise we can increase our overall food intake – including micronutrients, antioxidants and other healthy plant-based compounds.

Exercise also promotes muscle development, for which protein is required – another reason to ensure you maintain an adequate daily intake of protein. A person with a higher proportion of muscle in their body is likely to have a higher metabolic rate – the rate at which they burn calories.[7] Exercise, therefore, reduces the prospect of weight gain in multiple ways. Exercise also offers holistic health benefits, including maintaining a healthy outlook, rebalancing body systems and (if exercising outdoors) helping us connect with nature.

Protein powder and processed supplements have deliberately not been included in these recipes. There are a few reasons for this. Firstly, protein powder and supplements are often heavily processed, and we prefer to use ingredients as close to their natural state as possible. The texture of protein powder can negatively impact the experience of eating the dish, and protein powder is also often more expensive than other sources of plant protein. On the other hand, protein powder is extremely high in protein, low in fat and carbohydrates, and it is extremely convenient – especially to add to smoothies and to make 'energy snacks', for example. You can add protein powder to many of these recipes to further increase the protein content.

These recipes are intended to enthuse and inspire you. Try them and create your own variations – there is so much more that is possible. Consider the recipes in this book as blueprints, waiting for you to come and make them your own. We hope you have lots of fun trying them out!

Consider the recipes in this book as blueprints, waiting for you to come and make them your own.

---

[6] Health Direct, *High fibre foods and diet*, Health Direct website, accessed November 2020. https://www.healthdirect.gov.au/high-fibre-foods-and-diet

[7] K Gunnars, *Protein intake – how much protein should you eat per day?*, Healthline website, accessed November 2020. https://www.healthline.com/nutrition/how-much-protein-per-day

Cooking temperature and equipment

The cooking temperatures are approximated and stated as 'high', 'medium' or 'low'. Baking temperatures are stated in degrees Celsius (°C). Be sure to monitor your food at all times when cooking. There is a conversion chart for cooking temperatures for your reference provided in the Resources section on page 161.

This book contains many cooking methods, including boiling, steaming, grilling, baking and sautéing. The latter deserves a special mention.

Sautéing requires cooking on high heat in a small amount of oil until the food starts to turn colour. This helps to release the flavour of the food into the dish. For the recipes in this book, a non-stick pan must be used to prevent food burning on the bottom of the pan. These recipes often call for you to sauté onion, garlic and spices – but vegetables and grains may also be cooked in this way. 'Sauté' is taken from the French verb *sauter* (to jump) because you need to stir and turn the food in the pan as it cooks.

A blender is indispensable – for blending raw ingredients, soups and smoothies. A small, powerful blender or food processor that can blend nuts and seeds, ginger and spices is useful. Other useful appliances include a rice cooker or steamer, oven or air-fryer, grill, pressure cooker and a stovetop and non-stick pans.

A garlic press to crush garlic and a grater to grate fresh ginger are useful, as well as sieves and a measuring jug.

Another appliance we highly recommend is a soy milk maker (see 'Home-made soy milk blend' on page 158).

A spice bag can be helpful for infusing the flavours of star anise, cardamom, clove pods and other whole spices, as it is easy to remove the bag from the dish when it is cooked.

A spice bag can be helpful for infusing the flavours of spices.

Weights and measures

Weights and measures are provided in cups and spoons or grams (g) or millilitres (ml) for liquids. A conversion chart is provided in the Resources section on page 161.

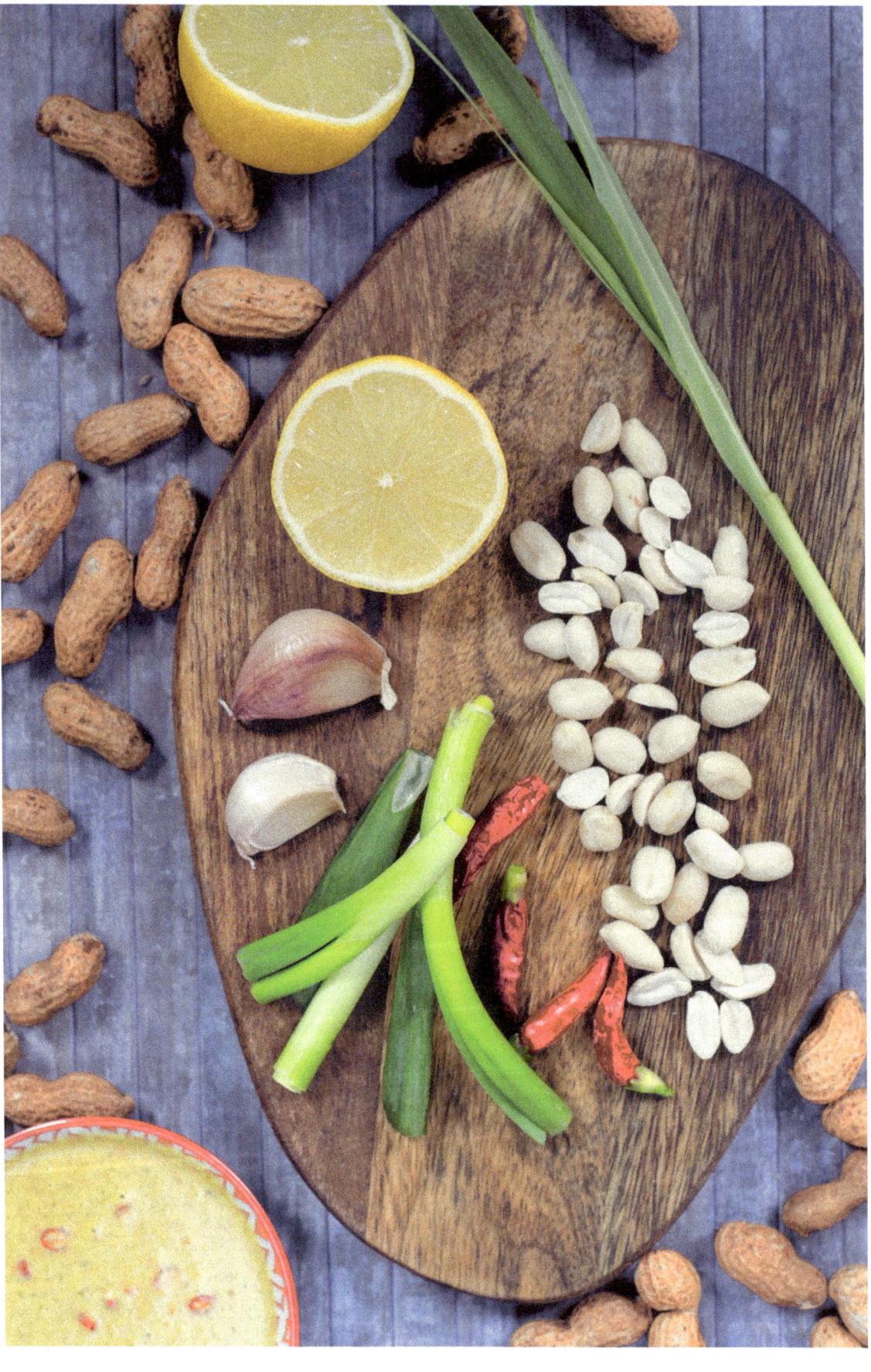

PANTRY LIST

A general rule of thumb is to use a 'little of everything' to ensure that your diet contains a balance of all the macro- and micronutrients that your body needs. Some of the key staple ingredients used in this book are described here for your reference.

Seasonal and regional

Where fruit and vegetables have been suggested it is usually possible to substitute these for seasonal fruit and vegetables that are available locally. In-season fruit and veggies are likely to be fresher and cheaper, and buying them is a good way to support local producers. Look out for organic options at your local farmers' markets – fresh fruit and vegetables that are grown without pesticides and not packaged in plastic are better for your health and more ecologically sustainable.

Look out for organic fruit and veggies at your local farmers' markets.

Spices, salt and seasoning

The potency of spices varies surprisingly widely depending on the variety purchased, how fresh the spice is, whether it's whole (e.g. pods) or ground and how it has been stored. It's preferable to buy whole spices in small quantities so that you can grind them just before using. Garlic can be crushed using a garlic press, and fresh ginger can be peeled and grated, or both can be blended in a small blender.

Quantities for salt have not been specified in most recipes as we prefer to leave it up to you to determine according to taste. Your healthcare provider may have advised you to consume less salt. At first, reducing salt intake seems difficult. However, most people find that as they start eating food with less salt their sense of taste adjusts. We recommend iodised salt for daily cooking – as many other sources of iodine are not available in a vegan-friendly diet.[8] Some recipes call for black salt (see page 9).

Oils

We recommend EVOO, coconut and avocado oil with high smoke points for cooking on high heat, supplemented with nut, hemp and flax-seed oils for salads.

Sweetener, sugar and the alternatives

With many new low-calorie alternatives to sugar now in our shops, you have the option of sweetening your desserts without significantly increasing the calories. An excellent zero-calorie option is stevia, a natural sweetener made from the leaves of the stevia plant.

If you do choose to use sugar, beet sugar is a good option as it is a product of sustainable farming techniques and vegan-friendly production (unlike white cane sugar). There are other vegan-friendly natural sweeteners such as maple syrup, molasses, malt extract, brown rice or sorghum syrup, coconut or monkfruit sugar and organic raw or unrefined cane sugar. Dates and fruits also make great sources of natural sweetness because they also contain vitamins and minerals.

We have taken a mixed approach in this book, principally using dates, malt extract and stevia. You can easily replace the stevia in our recipes with one of the sugars or natural sweeteners recommended above. You will need to adjust the nutritional information for your choice of sugar or sweetener. Raw caster sugar, for example, will add approximately 11 calories per teaspoon of sugar to your calorie intake.

You may also choose to adjust the amount of sugar or sweetener in the dessert recipes according to your taste. If you commit to consuming less sugar in your diet, your sense of taste will gradually adjust. You will find that the natural flavours of your food start to come through more and more as your palate adjusts to lower sugar levels.

We recommend stevia or organic, vegan-friendly sugars or natural sweeteners.

---

8   Health Direct, *Iodine*, Health Direct website, accessed November 2020. https://www.healthdirect.gov.au/iodine

There are a few ingredients that you will need frequently, and we suggest stocking up on these to make the most of the recipes. They are chosen for their nutritional content as well as their taste.

Almonds

Almonds are packed with vitamin E and healthy fats. They also taste really good! We use almonds sparingly as their high-fat content gives them their high calorific value. However, they are perfect in small quantities.

Beans, seeds and legumes

Used throughout this book, beans, seeds and legumes such as peas, lentils and chickpeas not only provide a source of protein but other nutrients as well. To ensure the nutrients are released to their full potential, soak raw beans, nuts, sunflower seeds and legumes overnight then rinse thoroughly before cooking. Check that your beans and legumes are properly cooked before serving to ensure they are easily digestible. Some beans – especially kidney beans – can be harmful if consumed before they are fully cooked. Soaking serves the secondary purpose of reducing cooking times. A pressure cooker will also reduce cooking times. If you don't have time to soak and cook your beans and legumes you can use tinned options instead.

Black salt – Himalayan

Available from some health food and Indian grocery stores, Himalayan black salt has a special flavour – if you can't source it go ahead and use regular salt. Note there are two kinds of black salt – be sure to buy the 'Himalayan' black salt, also called 'kala namak' or 'Indian black salt'.

Carrots and sweet potatoes

Carrots and sweet potatoes, especially the red and purple varieties, are two exceptional vegetables.

Carrots and sweet potatoes, especially the red and purple varieties, are two exceptional vegetables in terms of both nutrition and taste. They provide vegan-friendly sources of vitamin A, as well as other important micronutrients and antioxidants. Sweet potatoes have a lower glycaemic index (GI) score (see page 15) than white or red potatoes and are therefore great staples for a vegan diet.

Chia seeds

We like to keep a jar of chia seeds handy for desserts. They look attractive and are high in micronutrients like calcium, manganese, magnesium, phosphorous and antioxidants. Chia seeds also contain omega-3 fatty acids. They swell up to 10 times their volume when in water, so check that they are fully hydrated before eating to avoid stomach upset.

Cocoa powder and cocoa nibs – FairTrade

High in potassium, calcium, iron and antioxidants, cocoa is just amazing – use in smoothies or high-protein desserts (be sure to look up the recipe for our chocolate dessert on page 143). To support sustainable farming businesses we recommend choosing brands that are certified 'FairTrade'.[9]

Coconut flour

Coconut flour is high fibre and gluten free. It has a sweet taste so keep it handy for sweets and desserts, though it can also be used in savoury dishes.

Desiccated coconut (ground or flakes)

Rich in manganese, copper and iron, desiccated coconut is great added to smoothies and as a dessert topping.

Flaxseed (also known as linseed)

A staple for a vegan diet, ground flaxseed is high in omega-3 fatty acids. Flaxseed can be ground just before using to get the full nutritional value. Ground flaxseed is often used as an egg replacement, by mixing 1 tablespoon ground flaxseed with 2½ tablespoons water. Let it stand for 5 minutes before using. Due to its nutritional content, it is also a key ingredient in our 'Seasonal coconut almond oat smoothie' recipe on page 150.

For the best-quality produce and to support sustainable agriculture we recommend choosing brands that are certified Fair Trade.

---

9   More information on FairTrade-certified brands for Australia and New Zealand is available at FairTrade Australia New Zealand website https://fairtradeanz.org.

Hemp seeds and hemp oil

Hemp seeds are high in methionine-containing protein, vitamin E, B vitamins including niacin, riboflavin, thiamine, vitamin B6 and folate and minerals. Hemp seeds and hemp oil also contain an optimal ratio of omega-3 to omega-6 fatty acids.[10]

Kiwi fruit

Kiwi fruits (especially the green variety) are particularly high in vitamins C, E, A and K and other immune-boosting compounds. We like to include one kiwi fruit a day in our diet and it is a tangy ingredient in the 'Green smoothie' recipe on page 153.

Malt extract

Malt extract is often included in recipes for its nutritional qualities as well as its taste. It's a particularly good source of B vitamins. Many sources of B vitamins are from animals and our bodies cannot store B vitamins (except for vitamin B12), so mindfully including sources of B vitamins is important for a plant-based diet. You can also substitute malt extract with molasses in many recipes.

Mirin

Mirin is a sweet rice wine originating from Japan. It is really easy to mistakenly get 'mirin seasoning' products from the supermarket that mimic real mirin. If you can't source genuine mirin feel free to substitute with apple juice or sweet soy sauce instead for the recipes in this book.

Miso

Miso is a fermented paste made from soybeans originating from Japan. It is available in several varieties and is stocked by most supermarkets. Check the ingredients on the packet to make sure your product is pure miso (with no added ingredients other than the soybeans and the starter culture).

Malt extract is often included in recipes for its nutritional qualities as well as its taste.

[10] Medical News Today, *Nutritional benefits*, Medical News Today website, accessed November 2020, https://www.medicalnewstoday.com/articles/323037#nutritional-benefits

Mushrooms

Mushrooms are loaded with B vitamins, selenium and antioxidants, which can be hard to obtain with a plant-based diet. The white button variety contains one of the non-animal sources of vitamin D (you can also get vitamin D from sunlight).

Nutritional yeast flakes

Nutritional yeast is a major vegan-friendly source of vitamin B12. Usually found in animal products, B12 is stored in the body and is vital for good health.

Olive oil – extra-virgin (EVOO)

Olive oil is one of the healthiest fats and is high in antioxidants which can help prevent cell damage in the body.[11] Extra-virgin olive oil (EVOO) is considered the healthiest as the oil is extracted using natural methods. Make sure you buy yours from a reputable source. If you don't have EVOO, hemp-seed oil (see page 11), grape-seed oil or a good-quality vegetable oil can be substituted. A spray nozzle for your oil is perfect to help cover larger surfaces with less oil – especially when baking.

Seaweed

Seaweed can be purchased fresh or dried and then rehydrated. Different types of seaweed have different nutrient profiles. Common varieties that can be purchased as dried products include *kombu*, *wakame* and *nori*. Importantly, they are all vegan-friendly sources of iodine and methionine. Iodine is essential to the function of the thyroid gland whilst methionine is an essential amino acid and complements the amino acid profiles of tofu and tempeh.

Sesame seeds

Sesame seeds are a great source of healthy fats, B vitamins, methionine, minerals, fibre, antioxidants and other compounds – and they taste really good! It is easy to get a lot of flavour

Olive oil is one of the healthiest fats and is high in antioxidants.

---

[11] Better Health Channel, *Antioxidants*, Better Health Channel website, accessed December 2020, https://www.betterhealth.vic.gov.au/health/healthyliving/antioxidants

suitable for both savoury and sweet dishes from a small number of seeds. Available as both black and white varieties, we recommend toasting them in batches and storing them in an airtight jar to use as sprinkles and toppings – they will keep for three to six months in your pantry.

Soy sauce ('light' soy sauce and 'sweet' soy sauce)

This book regularly uses both light soy sauce and sweet soy sauce. These can be found in Asian groceries and some supermarkets. Be sure to check the ingredients – your light soy sauce should not contain sugar. Sweet soy sauce can be labelled as 'kecap manis'. Opt for high-quality brands that use few additives – and check there are no added fish products (like 'bonita' or shrimp) for vegan-friendly choices.

Spinach

Spinach is a nutrient-loaded vegetable and eating a daily portion ensures you get a hearty dose of potassium, vitamins A and E, iron, folate and calcium every day alongside other micronutrients and antioxidants. We consider spinach a staple food for a vegan diet.

Sunflower seed kernels

Like almonds, sunflower seed kernels are packed with vitamin E. As with vitamin A, your body can store vitamin E. However, you need to maintain levels of these over time. Sunflower seeds are also high in selenium, zinc and flavonoids.

Like almonds, sunflower seed kernels are packed with vitamin E.

Soybeans and soy milk

We make our own soy milk blend and we highly recommend doing this. One of the best investments you can make is a consumer-grade soy-milk maker. On page 158 you will find a recipe that combines the goodness of soybeans, almonds and sunflower seeds.

If you are purchasing soy milk from the store, be sure to check the ingredients especially the added ingredients that can change the nutrient profile. 'Light' soy milk options are usually the best. Soy milk can be an important natural source of calcium for a vegan diet, so be sure to check the calcium content if you routinely substitute soy milk with other alternative kinds of milk.

Sweetener – stevia

Stevia, an extract from the stevia plant, is available in different forms including granules and liquid. We use stevia granules in this book. You can substitute stevia with the sweetener of your choice – remember to check and adjust the nutritional information for the recipe.

Tempeh (or 'tempe')

Tempeh is a product that is usually sold in blocks of approximately 250–300g and is made by fermenting soybeans. It can be found in the refrigerated or frozen section of supermarkets and Asian grocery stores. You can make tempeh at home if you can source the starter agent and set up an area in your kitchen to maintain the correct temperature for the fermenting process.

With a nutty flavour, tempeh is rich in micronutrients including iron, calcium and B vitamins as well as prebiotics and other helpful plant compounds. The type of tempeh used in the recipes in this book is 'plain tempeh' or 'raw tempeh' rather than marinated tempeh.

Tofu

Tofu, which comes in many varieties, is made from soybeans, water and a coagulant. As with all plant-based foods, it requires fewer carbon emissions to produce than meat or dairy [12] and it is often substantially cheaper to buy. Tofu is high in protein and contains a complete amino acid profile. It also contains comprehensive omega-3 and omega-6 fatty acids, calcium and vitamin D.

Tofu is high in protein and contains a complete amino acid profile.

Many recipes in this book use 'firm tofu' or 'soft tofu'. Firm tofu can usually be substituted with 'extra-firm tofu'. There is also a 'semi-firm tofu' and a type that is extremely smooth called 'silken tofu' that is delicious eaten raw. For many recipes in this book 'silken tofu', 'semi-firm' and 'soft tofu' can be used interchangeably. Consistency does vary with the brand. With

---

[12] D Carrington, 'Avoiding meat and dairy is "single biggest way" to reduce your impact on earth', The Guardian website, accessed November 2020. https://www.theguardian.com/environment/2018/may/31/avoiding-meat-and-dairy-is-single-biggest-way-to-reduce-your-impact-on-earth

experience, you will come to know which brands you like best and which brands are available in shops near you.

The key to enjoying tofu is the marinade, a mix of herbs, spices and liquids in which you chill the tofu for several hours or overnight to infuse it with flavour. To inspire you we have included a whole section on marinades starting on page 105.

Textured vegetable protein (TVP) and soy chunks

TVP and soy chunks are more highly processed versions of soy with the fats totally removed. High in protein and low in fat, these are your top product choices for slimming. They are packaged as dried products and are therefore easy to store. TVP and soy chunks can be ridiculously cheap compared to other protein sources. On the downside, they are highly processed, and store-purchased products made with TVP or soy chunks are often high in fat and salt.

Vanilla essence – FairTrade

Vanilla essence is the extract from the vanilla bean and is used frequently in soy milk blends and desserts. We recommend choosing brands that are certified 'FairTrade' (see page 10).

Whole grains

Carbohydrates are broken down into sugars in our bodies. The type of carbohydrates we consume is important – sugars that dissolve quickly into the bloodstream can make your energy profile look like a roller coaster as your blood-sugar levels fluctuate through the day. In some people, this can contribute to binge eating when experiencing blood-sugar 'lows'. The glycaemic index (GI) measures the amount of sugar in a food and how quickly it is released into the bloodstream.[13] With a lower GI score, whole grains contain less readily available sugar, more fibre per gram and are considered more filling than the same quantity of processed grains. Choose whole grains to avoid the highs and lows of blood-sugar levels that starchy foods can cause.

Barley is an example of a low-GI grain, and we have included a few other whole grains in this book including millet, freekeh sorghum and amaranth.

Choose whole grains to avoid the highs and lows of blood-sugar levels that starchy foods can cause.

---

13   Health Direct, *Carbohydrates*, Health Direct website, accessed November 2020, https://www.healthdirect.gov.au/carbohydrates

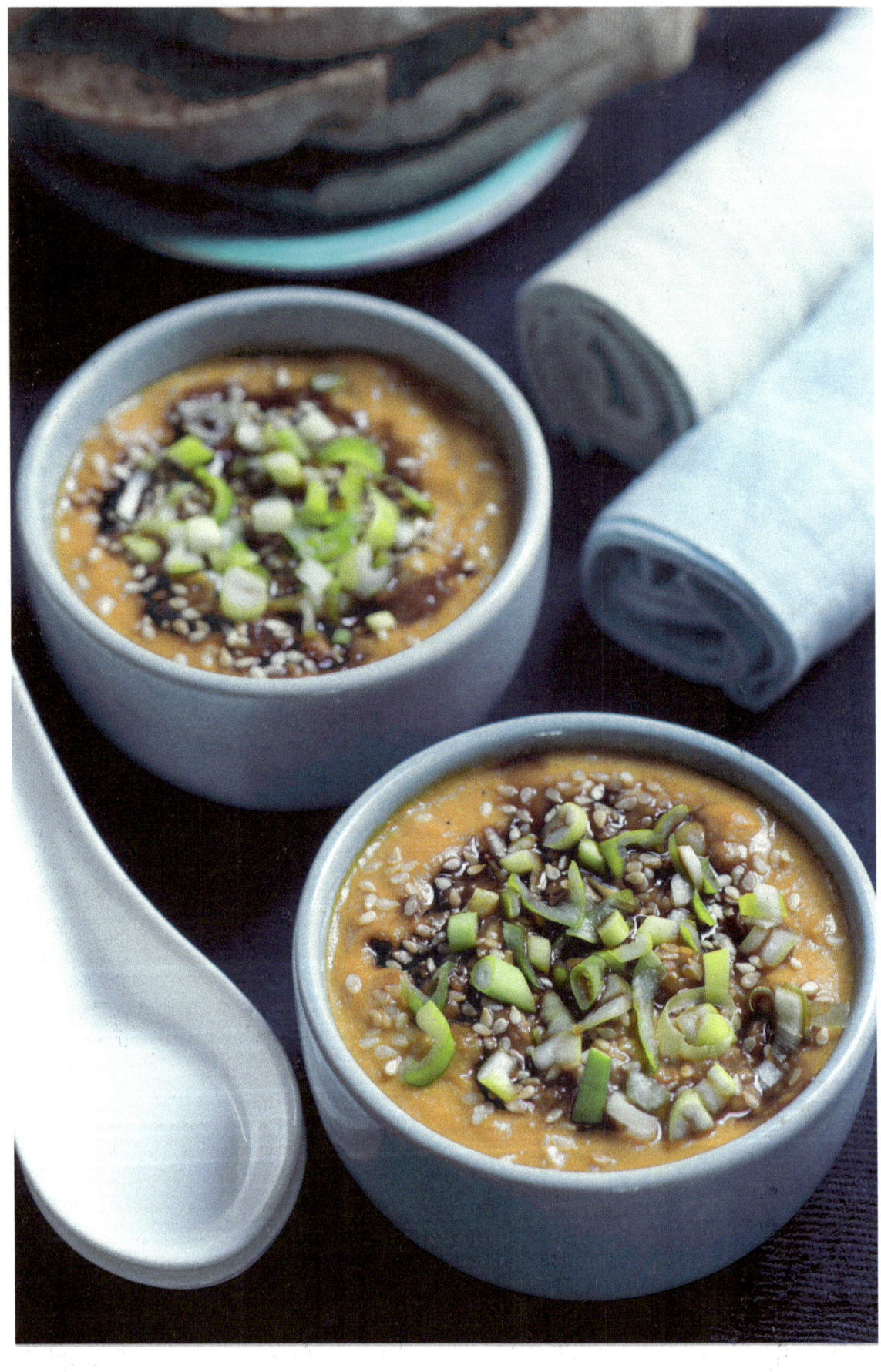

SOUPS

There's nothing more warming than a soup. This collection of soups has been created to inspire you using plant-based staples including spinach, mushroom and sweet potato.

It's easy to squeeze in some extra fibre in soups! The use of pearl barley in *'Sweet potato, ginger and barley soup'* on page 26 adds fibre and flavour to this high-protein soup.

The use of soft tofu in *'Sweet potato, pea and miso soup'* on page 29 creates a rich, creamy texture whilst providing a balanced nutritional profile loaded with protein.

Soups are the ideal way to use up leftover ingredients – go ahead and substitute the veggies with what you have in your refrigerator or pantry. Using up leftover food in soups is a great way to reduce food waste!

MUSHROOM SOUP

KCAL 160 | PROTEIN 9g | FAT 6.8g | CARBS 17g | SERVES 4

INGREDIENTS

350g mushrooms

2 onions

2 cloves garlic

1 tbsp extra-virgin olive oil

pinch of salt

pinch of black pepper

½ tsp thyme

2 cups light soy milk

2 cups vegetable stock

For the garnish

2 tbsp finely chopped fresh parsley

METHOD

1. Wash and finely chop the mushrooms, peel and finely chop the onions and crush the garlic.

2. Sauté the onions and garlic in the olive oil, salt and pepper. Add the mushrooms and thyme and cook for 1–2 minutes.

3. Add the light soy milk and vegetable stock and simmer on low heat for 2–3 minutes until tender.

4. Let the soup cool then add to a blender. Blend to the desired consistency.

5. Serve with parsley to garnish.

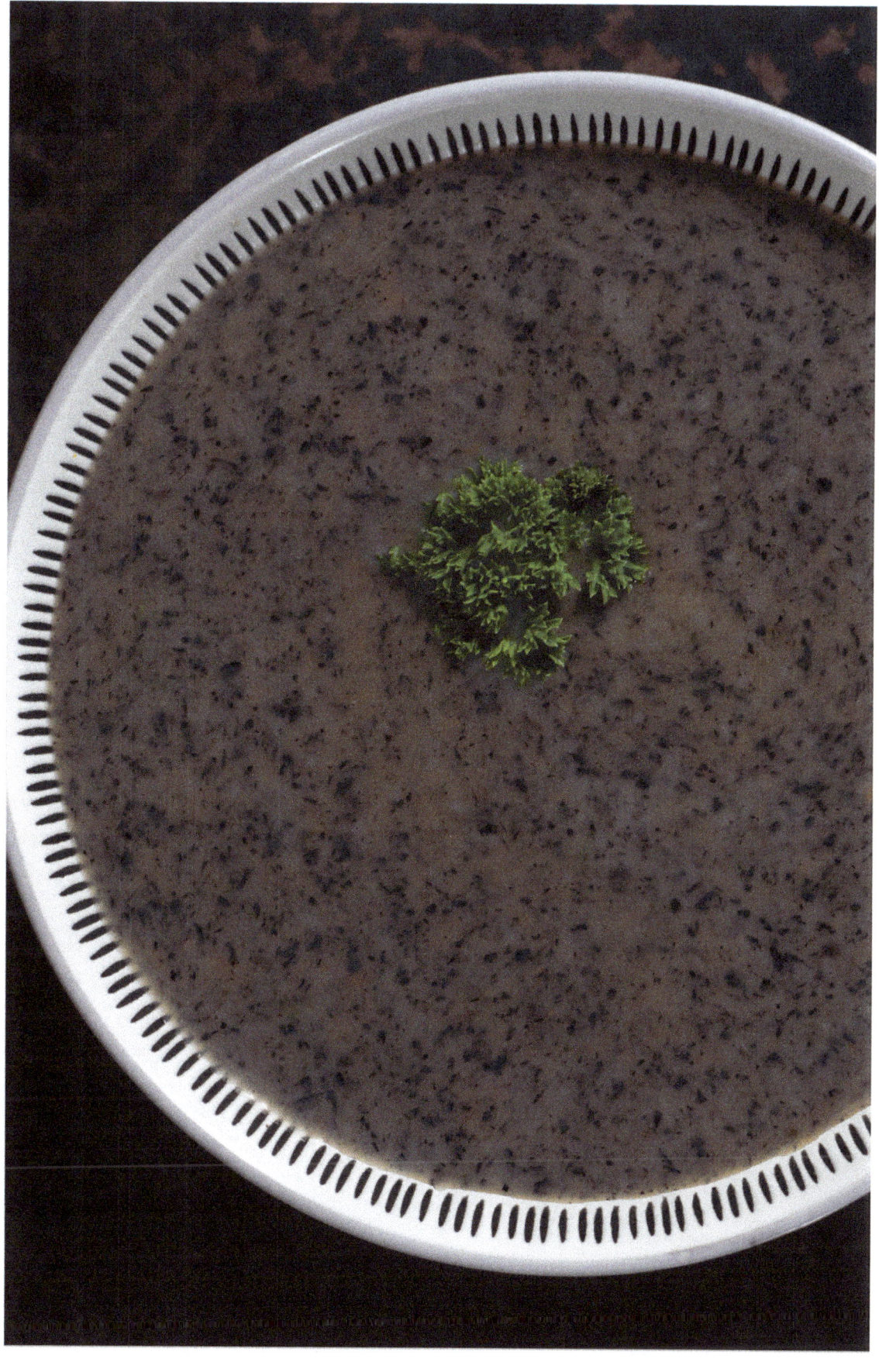

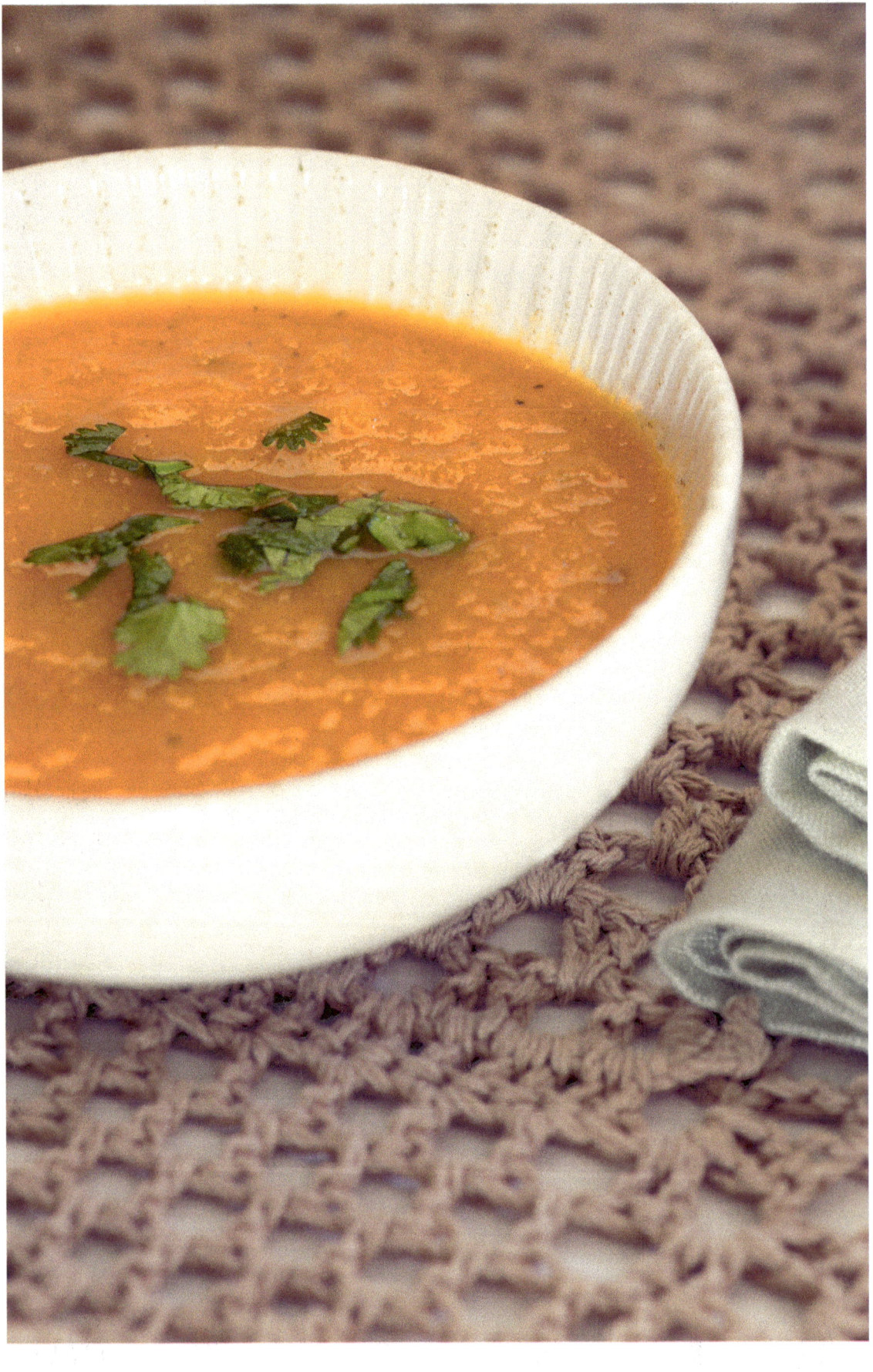

CARROT & CARAWAY SOUP

KCAL 98 | PROTEIN 3.3g | FAT 1.7g | CARBS 15g | SERVES 4

INGREDIENTS

1 sweet potato

4 carrots

2 sticks celery

1-inch stick ginger

2 cloves garlic

1 tbsp extra-virgin olive oil

½ tsp caraway seeds

4 tbsp nutritional yeast flakes

2 cups water

pinch of salt

pinch of black pepper

For the garnish

2 tbsp fresh herbs, chopped

METHOD

1. Peel and wash the vegetables and roughly chop.

2. Grate the fresh ginger and crush the garlic. Sauté in the olive oil until they change colour. Add the caraway seeds, vegetables, nutritional yeast, water and seasoning to taste.

3. Bring to the boil, place a lid on the pan and switch off the heat. Leave to cook for 15 minutes.

4. Wait for the mixture to cool slightly, then transfer the mixture to a blender. Blend to the desired consistency.

5. Garnish with fresh herbs to serve.

MISO & TOFU SOUP

KCAL 173 | PROTEIN 12g | FAT 4.1g | CARBS 28g | SERVES 2

INGREDIENTS

50g dried shiitake mushrooms

100g dried tofu

4 spring onions

1-inch stick ginger

1 bok choy (optional)

4 cups water

2 tbsp miso

2 tbsp light soy sauce

For the garnish

fresh coriander, chopped

METHOD

1. Soak the shiitake mushrooms and dried tofu overnight and retain the water. Wash and chop the spring onions and grate the ginger. If you are using bok choy, rinse and chop roughly.

2. Put the rinsed mushrooms and tofu together with the water in a pan with remaining ingredients except bok choy. Bring to the boil and let it simmer for 2–3 minutes.

3. If you are using bok choy add it to the pan and turn off the heat. Replace the lid and let it stand for 1 minute.

4. Serve garnished with freshly chopped coriander.

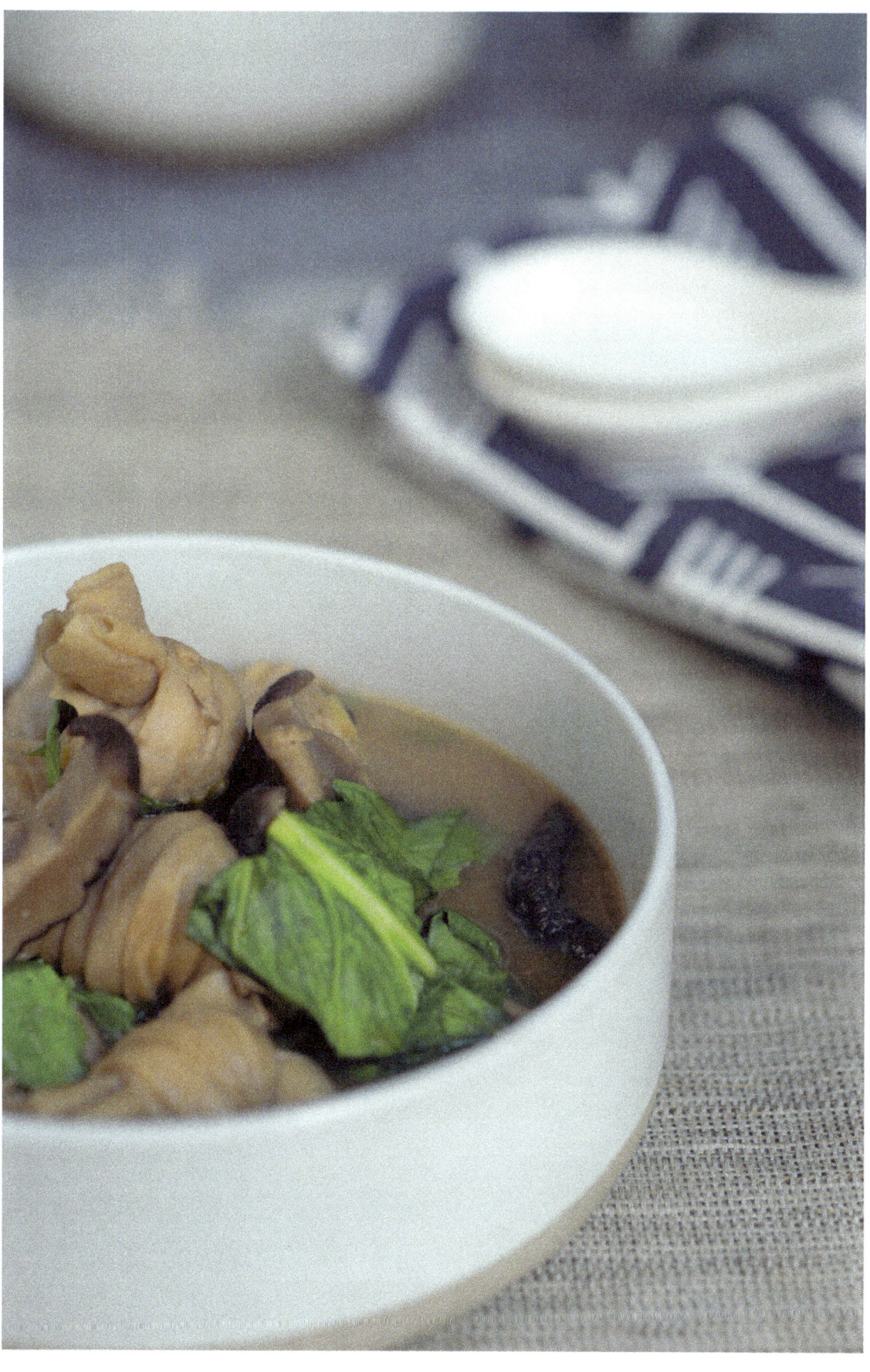

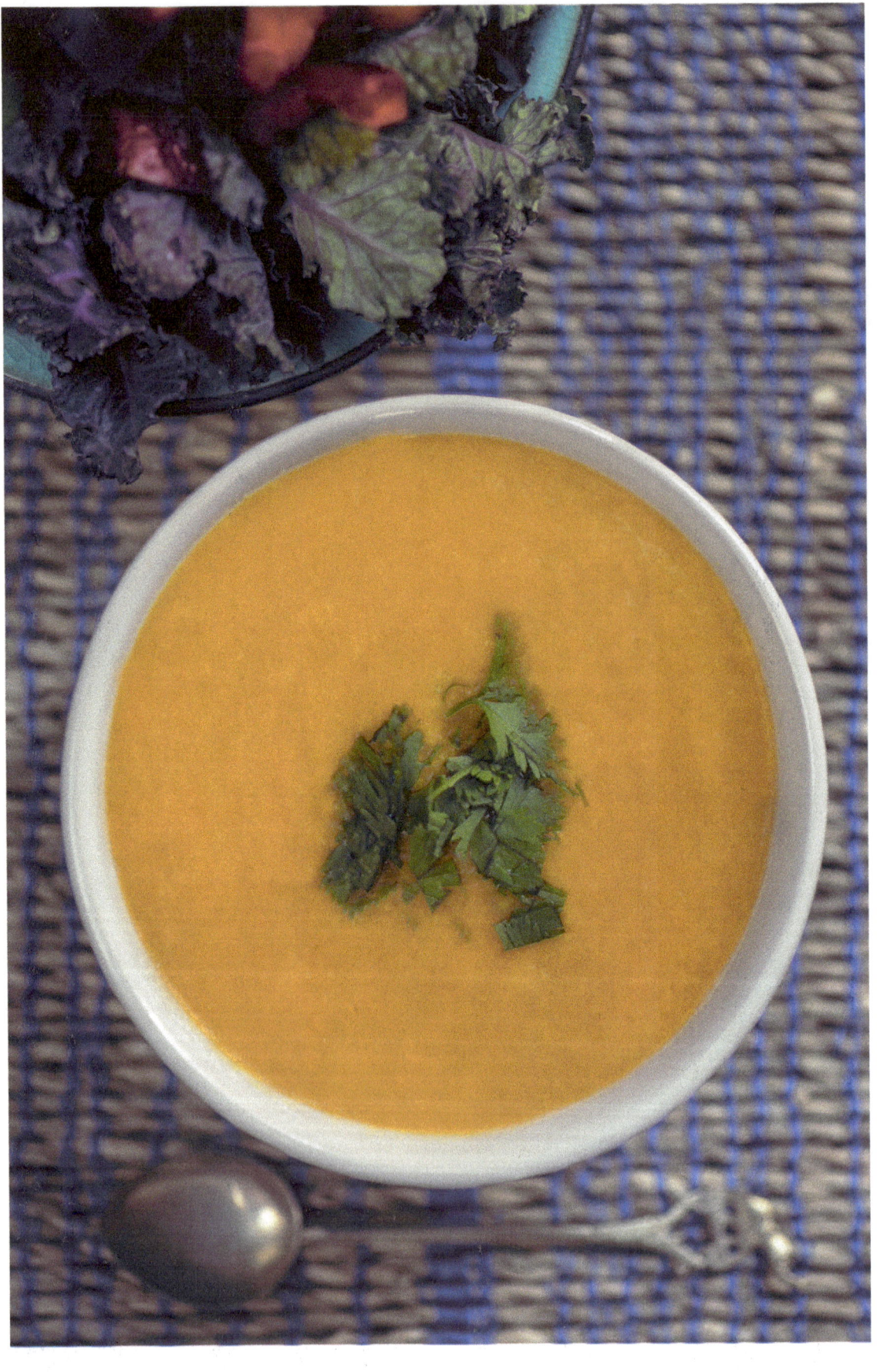

DAHL SOUP

KCAL 103 | PROTEIN 6.4g | FAT 1.6g | CARBS 19g | SERVES 4

INGREDIENTS

2 carrots

1 stick ginger

2 cloves garlic

¼ cup orange lentils

1 tsp extra-virgin olive oil

½ tsp cumin seeds

½ tsp turmeric

¼ tsp nutmeg

¼ tsp chilli powder

pinch of salt and black pepper or to taste

2 curry leaves (optional)

2 cups water

For the garnish

fresh coriander, chopped

METHOD

1. Wash, peel and roughly chop the carrots. Wash, peel and grate the ginger. Crush the garlic with a garlic press. Rinse and drain the lentils.

2. Sauté the garlic in the olive oil with the spices, curry leaves (if using), salt and pepper.

3. Add the lentils, water and carrots and bring to the boil. Simmer for 10–15 minutes or until the lentils are tender.

4. Allow the mixture to cool then add to a blender. Blend to the desired consistency.

5. Serve with fresh chopped coriander to garnish.

Note

1. Orange lentils are also called 'red lentils' or 'masoor dahl'.

SWEET POTATO, GINGER & BARLEY SOUP

KCAL 324 | PROTEIN 18g | FAT 15g | CARBS 36g | SERVES 4

INGREDIENTS

1 sweet potato

2 carrots

2 sticks celery

2 chilli peppers

1 small red capsicum (bell pepper)

¼ cup pearl barley

200g firm tofu, cubed

200g fried tofu, cubed (optional)

2 cloves garlic

2 sticks ginger

2 sticks galangal (optional)

1 tsp extra-virgin olive oil

½ tsp fennel seeds

pinch of salt

1 tbsp fresh lemon juice

To garnish

fresh coriander, chopped

METHOD

1. Wash, peel and thinly slice the sweet potato, carrots, celery, chillis and capsicum. Rinse and drain the pearl barley and tofu.

2. Grate the garlic, ginger and galangal (if using) or blend into a paste in a small blender. Sauté the mixture in the olive oil, add the pearl barley and fennel seeds. Cook for approximately 5 minutes or until the pearl barley starts to turn translucent.

3. Add all the remaining ingredients except the fresh coriander and bring to the boil. Simmer for 10 minutes or until the barley, potato and carrots are cooked.

4. Remove from heat and serve garnished with fresh coriander.

Notes

1. Fried tofu can be purchased from a store or you can make it at home. You can also use seitan, which is made from wheat gluten, as a substitute to add variety to your soup. The nutritional information will change according to the ingredients used.

2. Galangal is often available from Asian grocery stores and looks similar to fresh ginger or turmeric.

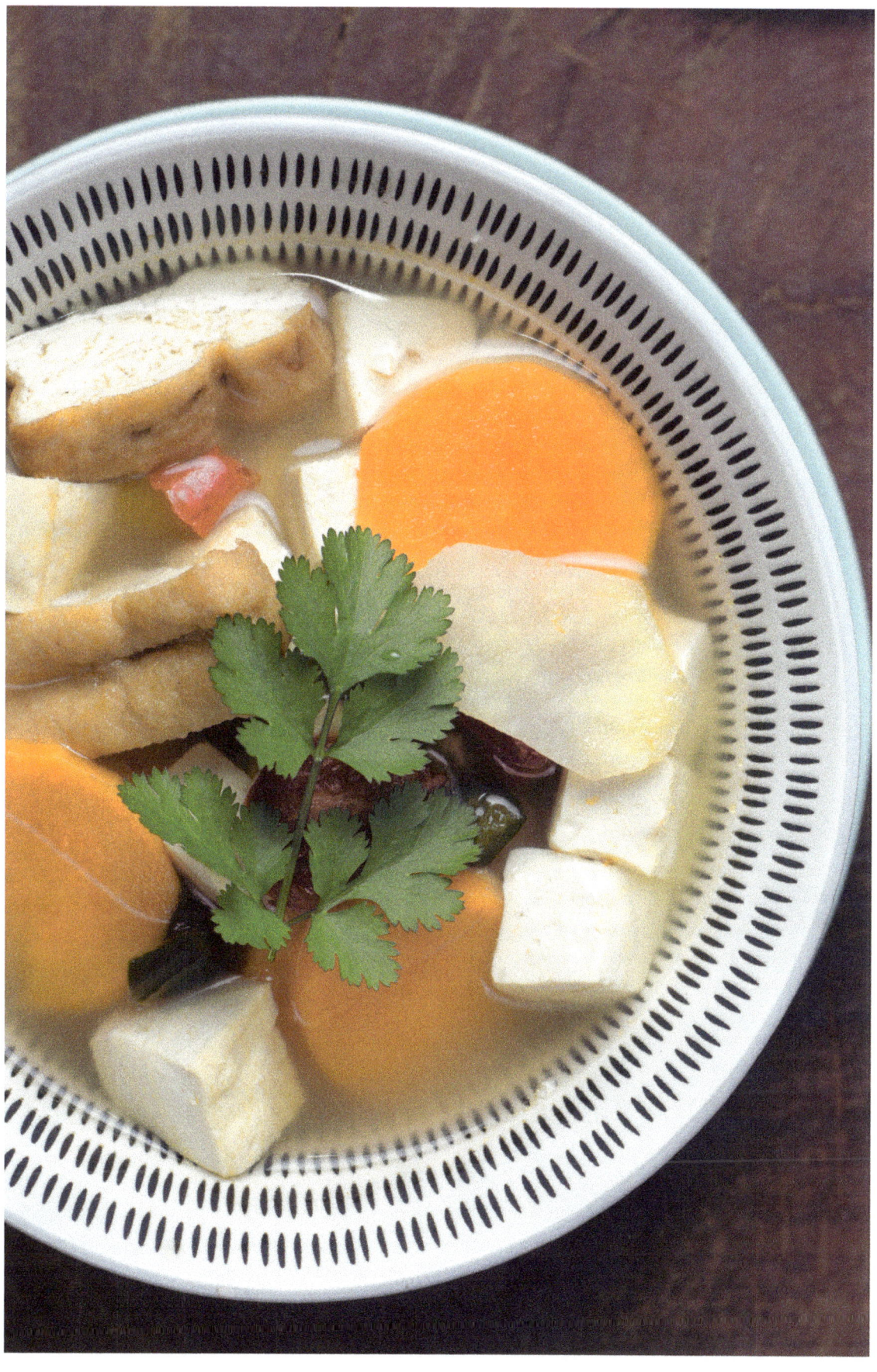

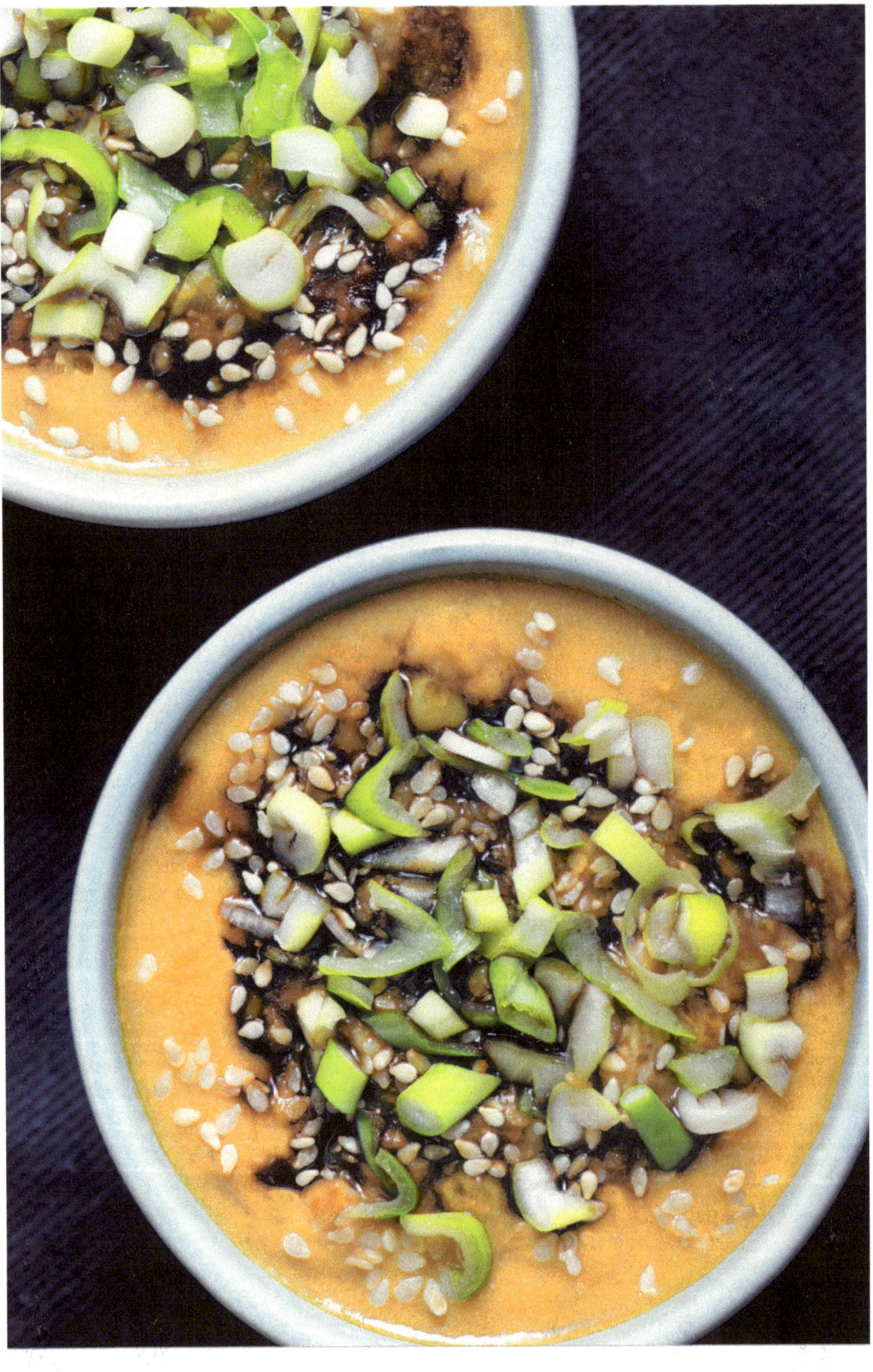

SWEET POTATO, PEA & MISO SOUP

KCAL 247 | PROTEIN 13g | FAT 6.4g | CARBS 38g | SERVES 4

INGREDIENTS

2 sweet potatoes

5 carrots

100g fresh peas

1 tsp miso

2 tbsp light soy sauce

1 tbsp sweet soy sauce

1 tbsp lemon juice

1 tbsp mirin

300g soft tofu

½ medium cucumber, peeled and chopped

For the garnish

fresh spring onions, finely chopped

2 tbsp sweet soy sauce

2 tbsp toasted sesame seeds

METHOD

1. Wash and roughly chop the sweet potatoes and carrots.

2. Steam or boil the sweet potatoes, carrots and peas. Set aside both the vegetables and the cooking water (stock) to cool slightly.

3. Blend the vegetable stock with the miso, soy sauces, lemon juice, mirin, soft tofu and cucumber. Add the vegetables, except the peas, and blend.

4. Stir in the peas.

5. Transfer to serving bowls and garnish with spring onion, soy sauce and toasted sesame seeds.

Note

1. You can substitute fresh peas with tinned peas and omit cooking them.

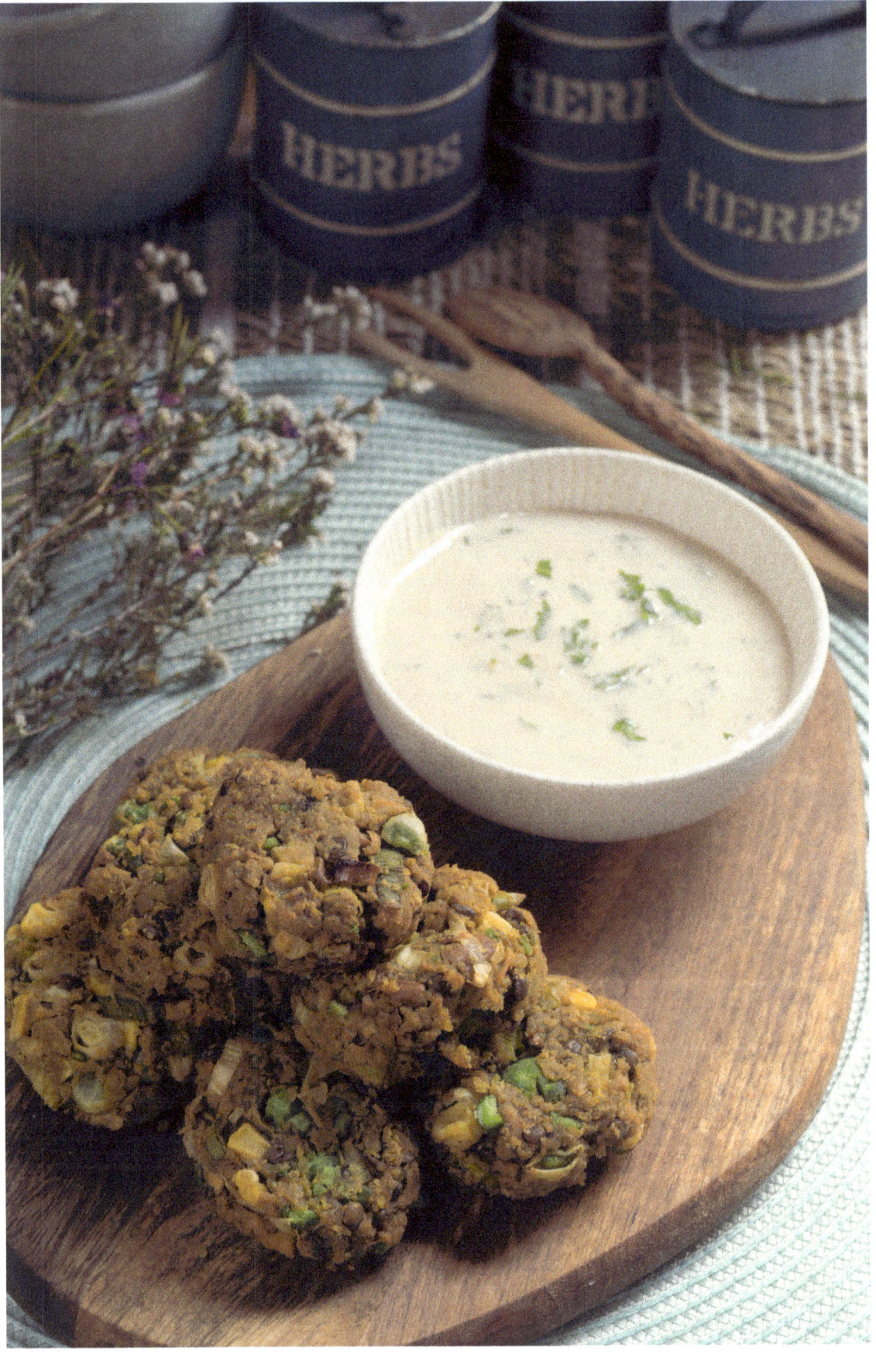

SNACKS & DIPS

Snacks are the perfect opportunity to maintain energy levels throughout the day – but watch out for the calories. Often we reach for high-fat and high-calorie chips and other snacks that don't really fill us up. This collection of snacks and dips provides ideas for high-protein alternatives so that you can maintain not only your energy levels but your protein levels as well.

There are also ideas for serving at parties and receptions, for example, the *'Roasted beetroot dip'* on page 44 and the *'Five bean oregano dip'* on page 32. The *'Hemp hummus and dough sticks'* on page 35 combines the goodness of sesame and chickpeas with hemp seeds to ensure a hearty dose of protein and micronutrients. The dough sticks are easy to make and are bound to impress!

Pair these snacks and dips with salads (beginning page 113) and dressings (beginning page 125).

FIVE BEAN OREGANO DIP

KCAL 169 | PROTEIN 9.1g | FAT 3.9g | CARBS 26g | SERVES 4

INGREDIENTS

80g cooked great northern beans

80g cooked pinto beans

80g cooked navy beans

80g cooked cannelloni beans

80g cooked butter beans

2 cloves garlic, crushed

1 stick ginger, peeled and grated

2 cloves garlic, crushed

1 tbsp extra-virgin olive oil

pinch of salt

pinch of black pepper

1 tbsp apple cider vinegar

¼ cup water

For the topping

freshly chopped oregano and parsley

METHOD

1. Sauté the garlic and ginger until the garlic starts to change colour. Add the beans and seasoning to the garlic and ginger paste, stir and cook for 1 minute.

2. Remove from the heat, let cool and add the apple cider vinegar. Place the mixture into a blender and add the water incrementally whilst blending.

3. Garnish with freshly chopped oregano and parsley to serve.

Notes

1. The beauty of this recipe is that it's an easy way to use up leftover cooked beans from the refrigerator. You can substitute the beans with different varieties (the nutritional value will vary slightly).

2. If cooking dried beans from scratch, this can take from 45 minutes up to 3 hours depending on the size and variety.

3. If you use dried kidney beans you must ensure they are fully cooked before using.

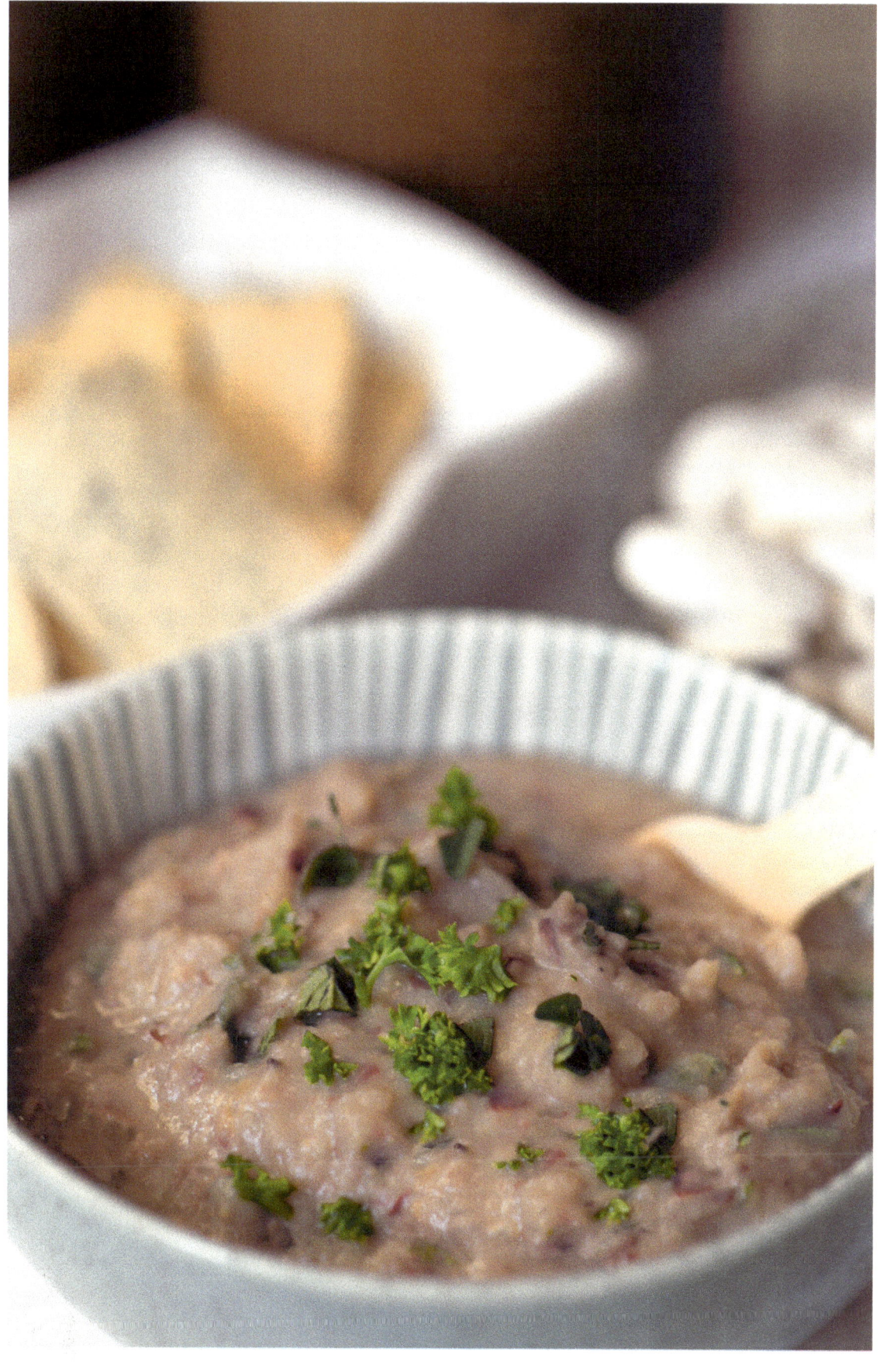

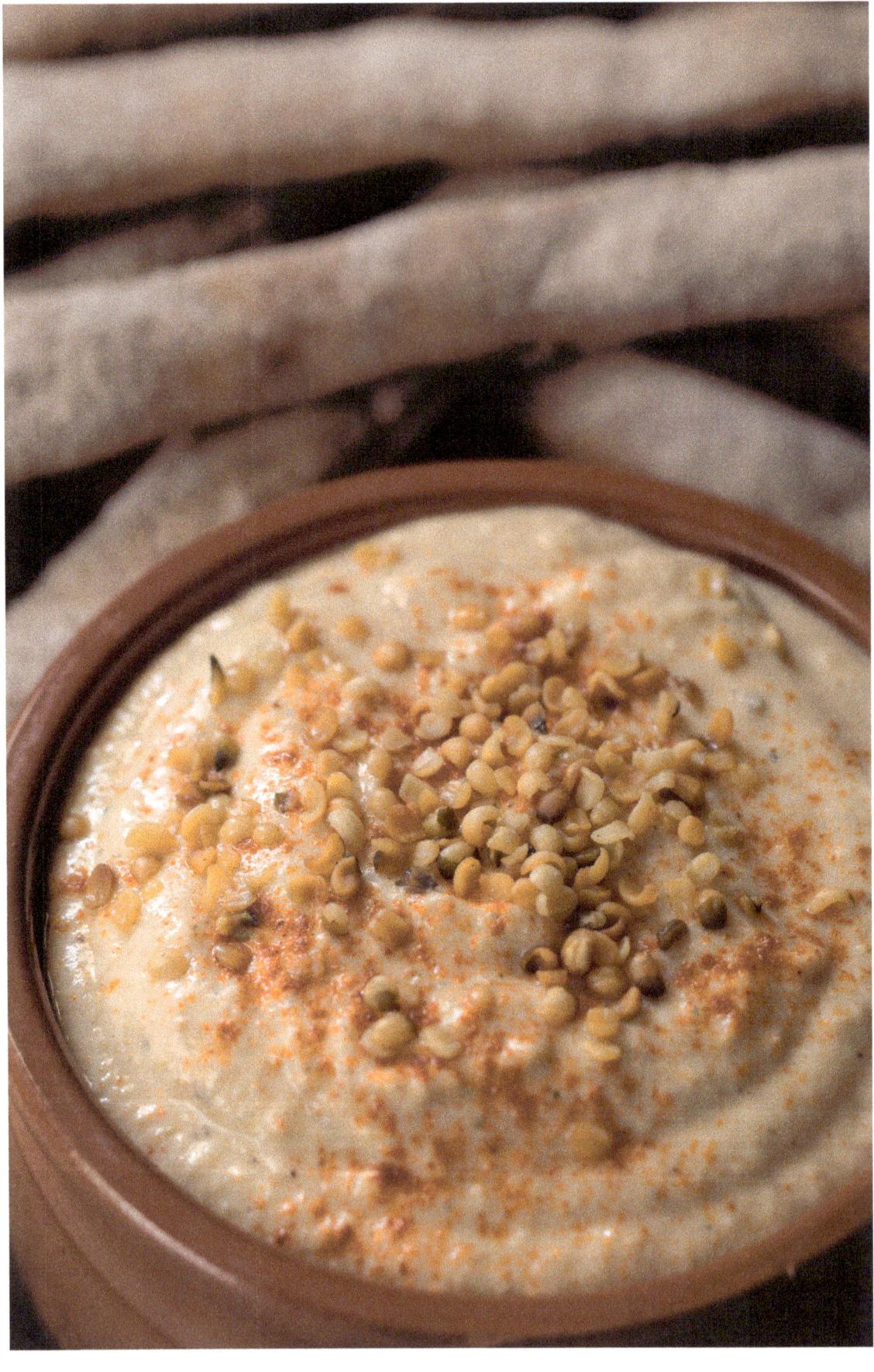

HEMP HUMMUS & DOUGH STICKS

KCAL 183 | PROTEIN 9.6g | FAT 7.1g | CARBS 23g | SERVES 10

INGREDIENTS

For the hummus

400g cooked chickpeas (or 175g dried chickpeas)

50g hemp seeds

2 tbsp tahini

2 cloves garlic

pinch of salt or to taste

¼ tsp white pepper

3 tbsp lemon juice

¼ tsp cumin powder

3 tbsp nutritional yeast flakes

¼ tsp paprika (optional)

½ cup water

For the dough sticks

1 sachet instant yeast

1⅔ cups spelt flour

¼ tsp garlic powder

2 tsp mixed Italian herbs

½ tsp thyme

pinch of salt or to taste

2 tbsp extra-virgin olive oil

½ cup warm water

METHOD

1. **For the hemp hummus (makes 10 servings)** – Rinse and drain the chickpeas. If using dried chickpeas, pre-soak, cook, rinse and drain. Spread the hemp seeds onto a baking tray and grill or toast in the oven on a low heat for 3–7 minutes or until they start to turn golden. Set aside and let cool.

2. Place all the ingredients except the water in a blender, setting some of the hemp seeds aside to use as a garnish. Add ¼ cup of the water and blend. Add water incrementally until your desired consistency is achieved.

3. Transfer to a storage pot or serving bowl and garnish with paprika powder (if using) and the remaining hemp seeds. Hemp hummus can be stored in the fridge for up to 3 days.

4. **For the dough sticks (makes 20 sticks, 2 sticks per serving)** – Mix the yeast sachet with the spelt flour and other dry ingredients in a large bowl. Make a well in the middle of the bowl and add 1 tbsp of the olive oil. Then add the warm water incrementally whilst mixing until a dough consistency is reached. Knead for 5 minutes then cover and leave to rise for 1 hour.

5. Roll the dough flat on a clean surface and cut into strips. Top with salt and brush or spray with 1 tbsp olive oil. Leave to rise for 1 more hour.

6. Bake for 10–15 minutes on medium heat or until the sticks start to turn golden. Allow to cool on a tray or wire rack before serving.

TOFU BITES

KCAL 243 | PROTEIN 21g | FAT 12g | CARBS 18g | SERVES 2

INGREDIENTS

300g extra-firm tofu

2 tbsp nutritional yeast flakes

½ tsp smoked paprika

1 tsp black salt (see note)

½ tsp black pepper

½ tsp ginger powder

1 tsp extra-virgin olive oil

3 tbsp fine polenta

1 tbsp cornflour

½ tsp mint, finely chopped

1 tsp Italian herbs

1 tbsp olive oil spray

For the marinade

1 tbsp sweet soy sauce

1 tbsp light soy sauce

1 tbsp apple cider vinegar

METHOD

1. **For the tofu** – Rinse and cut the tofu into cubes. Mix together the marinade ingredients and leave to marinate overnight.

2. **For the crumb** – Make a dry polenta herb crumb mix with remaining ingredients (except olive oil spray).

3. Drain the tofu, discarding the marinade. Coat the tofu cubes directly in the crumb mix. Arrange the cubes on a non-stick baking tray and spray lightly with oil.

4. Bake for 30 minutes on high, turning once.

5. Serve.

Note

1. If you don't have black salt you can substitute with regular salt.

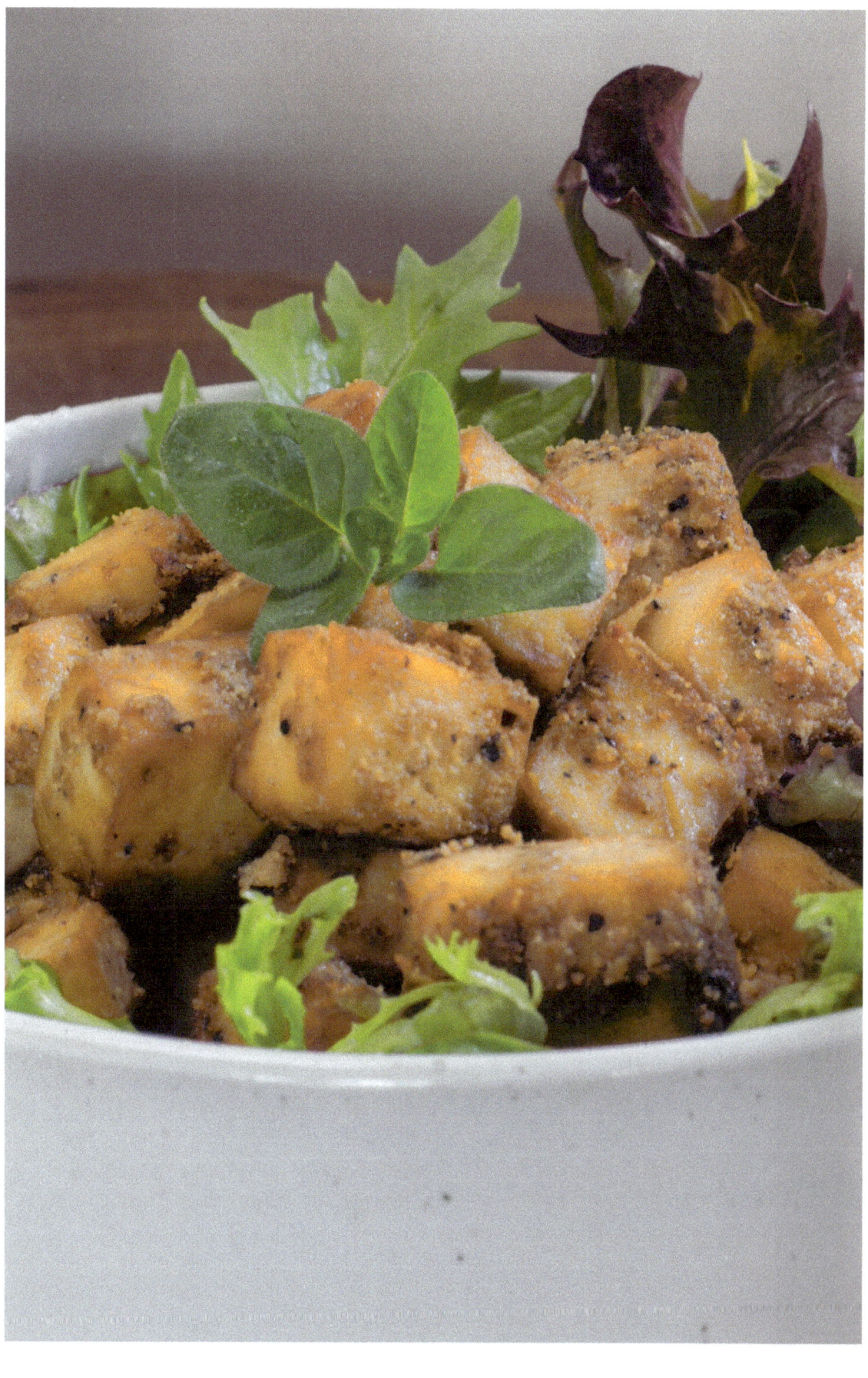

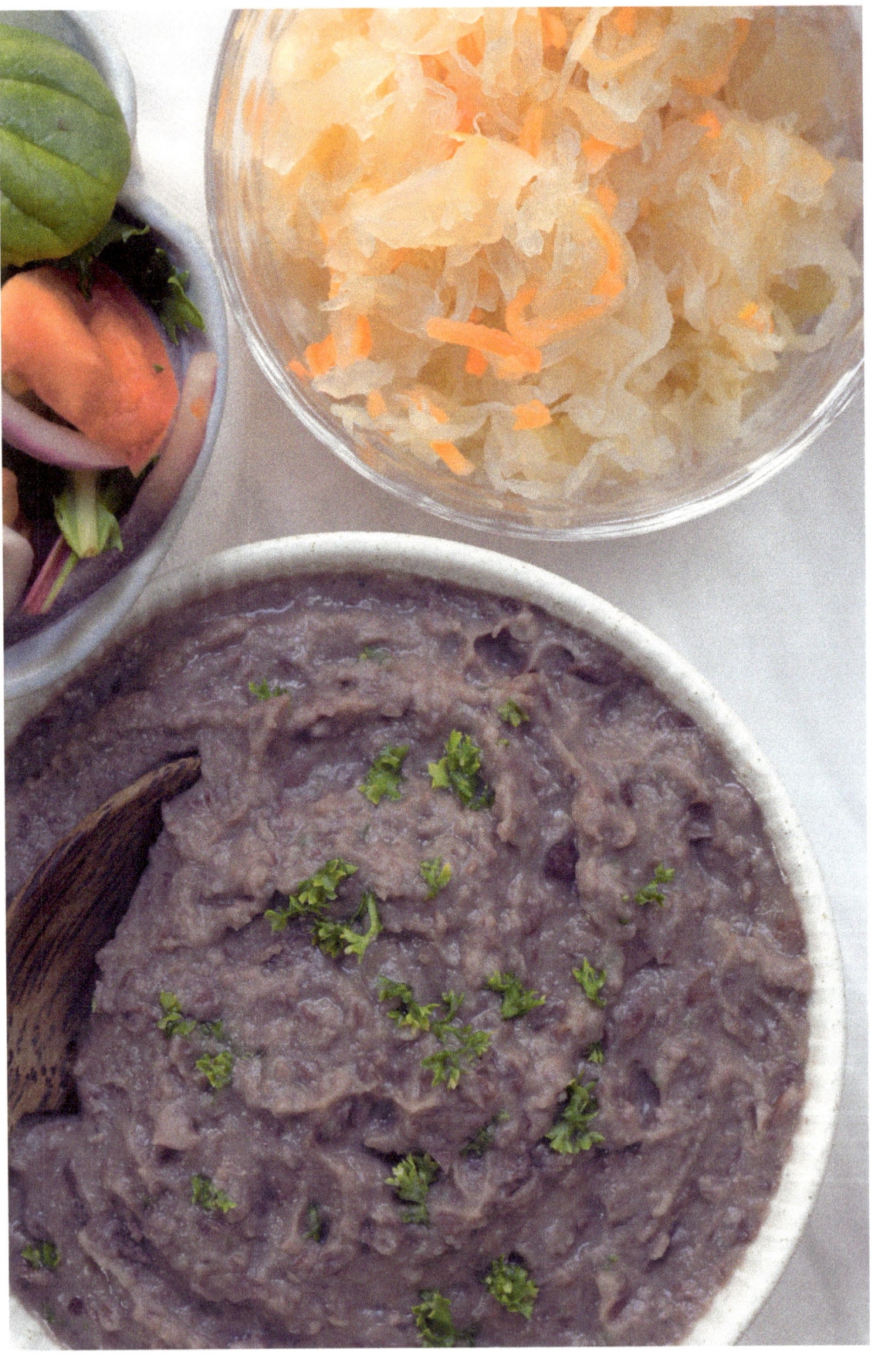

BLACK BEAN, LIME & CORIANDER DIP

KCAL 178 | PROTEIN 11g | FAT 1.3g | CARBS 32g | SERVES 8

INGREDIENTS

400g cooked black beans (or 150g dried black beans)

2 cloves garlic, crushed

2-inch stick ginger, peeled and grated

1 tbsp lime juice

1 tsp extra-virgin olive oil

pinch of salt

pinch of black pepper

¼ cup water

For the garnish

freshly chopped coriander

METHOD

1. Rinse and drain the beans. If using dried beans, pre-soak, cook, rinse and drain.

2. Sauté the garlic and ginger in the olive oil.

3. Add the beans and remaining ingredients except the water and cook for 1–2 minutes. Add the water and cook for another minute.

4. Remove from the heat and cool. Place the mixture in a blender and blend, adding more water as necessary to achieve desired consistency.

5. Place in a serving bowl and garnish with fresh coriander.

SPINACH HUMMUS

KCAL 90 | PROTEIN 5g | FAT 3.1g | CARBS 13g | SERVES 10

INGREDIENTS

200g fresh spinach

400g cooked chickpeas (or 175g dried chickpeas)

2 tbsp tahini

2 cloves garlic

2 tbsp lemon juice

pinch of salt

pinch of black pepper

¼ cup water plus more as needed

For the garnish

1 tbsp sesame seeds, toasted

1 tbsp sweet soy sauce

METHOD

1. Wash and drain the spinach thoroughly. Rinse and drain the chickpeas. If using dried chickpeas, pre-soak, cook, rinse and drain.

2. Place all the ingredients except the water in a blender. Add the water and blend, adding more water incrementally until the desired consistency is achieved.

3. Transfer to a storage pot or serving bowl and garnish with the sesame seeds and sweet soy sauce. Spinach hummus can be stored in the fridge for 2–3 days.

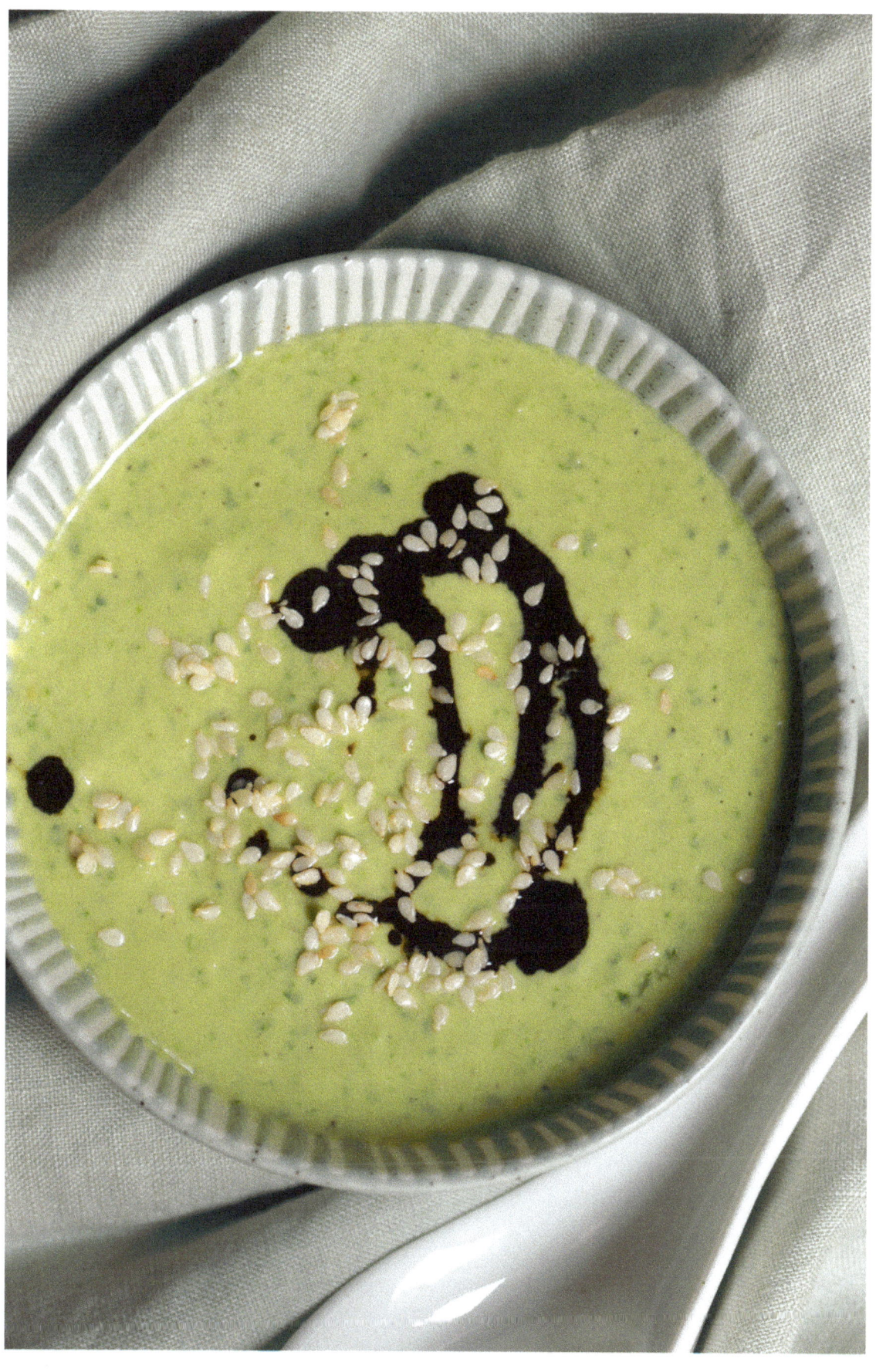

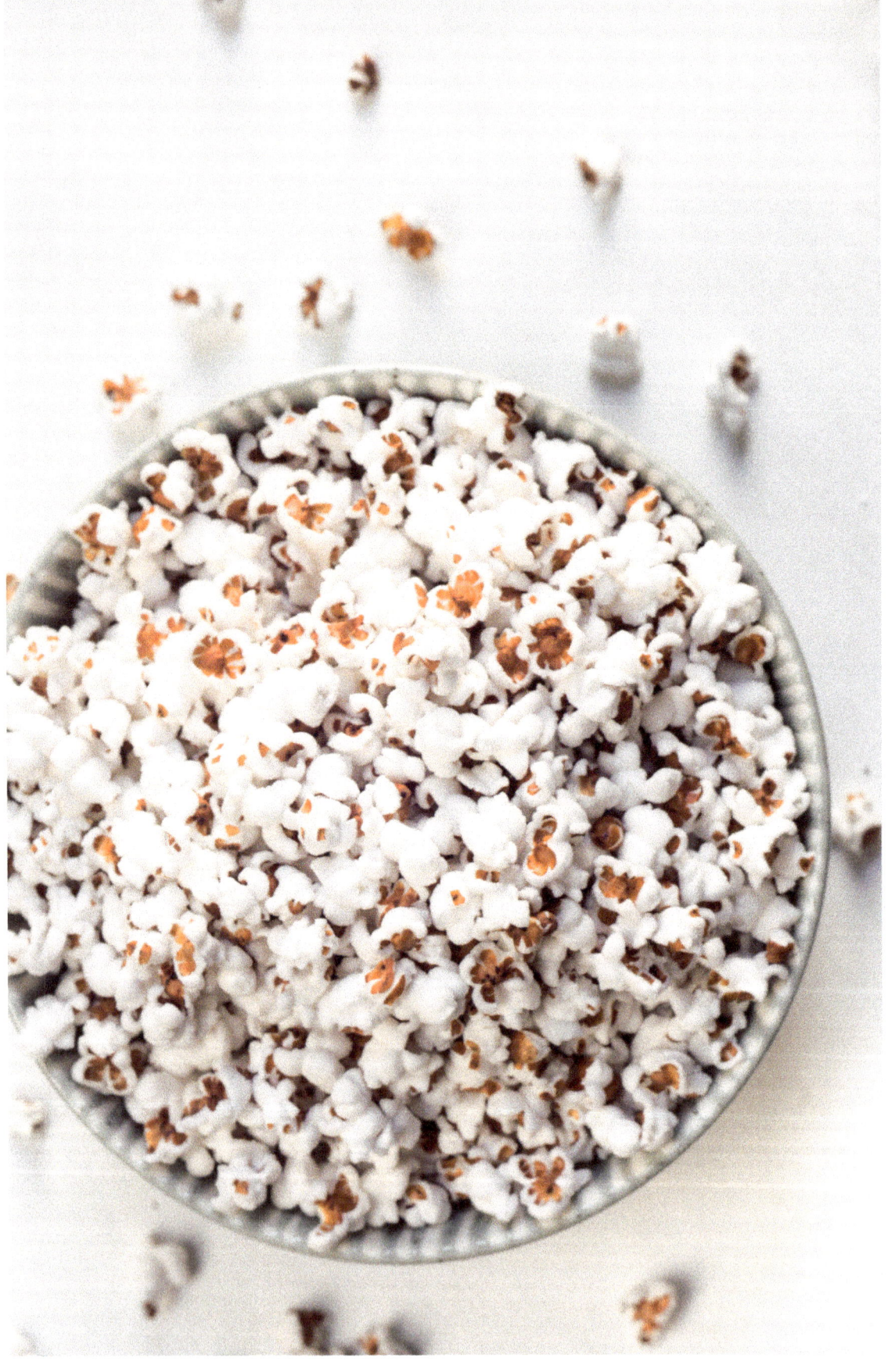

SORGHUM POPCORN

KCAL 59 | PROTEIN 3.4g | FAT 1.9g | CARBS 9g | SERVES 4

INGREDIENTS

3 tbsp sorghum grains
1 tsp extra-virgin olive oil
2 tbsp nutritional yeast flakes
pinch of salt
seasoning (optional – see note)

METHOD

1. Place the sorghum in a large saucepan with a lid and the olive oil.

2. Heat on medium-high heat. When the grains are hot enough they will start to pop. Keep the lid on until the popping noise subsides. Turn off the heat.

3. Add the yeast flakes, salt and any seasoning to a small blender and blend until fine. Add to the popcorn, shake well and serve.

Notes

1. It is *not* recommended to 'pop' sorghum in consumer popcorn machines designed to be used with maize kernels due to the difference in temperature at which the kernels pop.

2. You can substitute maize corn kernels instead of sorghum for traditional popcorn.

3. You can also mix in other seasoning such as smoked paprika or fine stevia granules, according to your taste.

ROASTED BEETROOT DIP

KCAL 56 | PROTEIN 4.1g | FAT 2.3g | CARBS 6.1g | SERVES 10

INGREDIENTS

500g beetroot

1 red onion

1 tsp extra-virgin olive oil

pinch of salt

300g soft or silken tofu

1 tsp paprika

1 tbsp lemon juice

pinch of black pepper

¼ cup soy milk

METHOD

1. Peel the beetroot and slice lengthwise. Slice the red onion and arrange with the beetroot on a baking tray. Spray lightly with the olive oil and sprinkle with salt. Roast in the oven on medium heat for 15–20 minutes or until the beetroot is cooked. Set aside and allow to cool.

2. When the vegetables are cooled transfer to a blender with remaining ingredients and blend until smooth.

3. Transfer the mixture to a small serving dish. Refrigerate to set and serve.

Note

1. Beetroot dip can be kept in an airtight container in the fridge for 2–3 days.

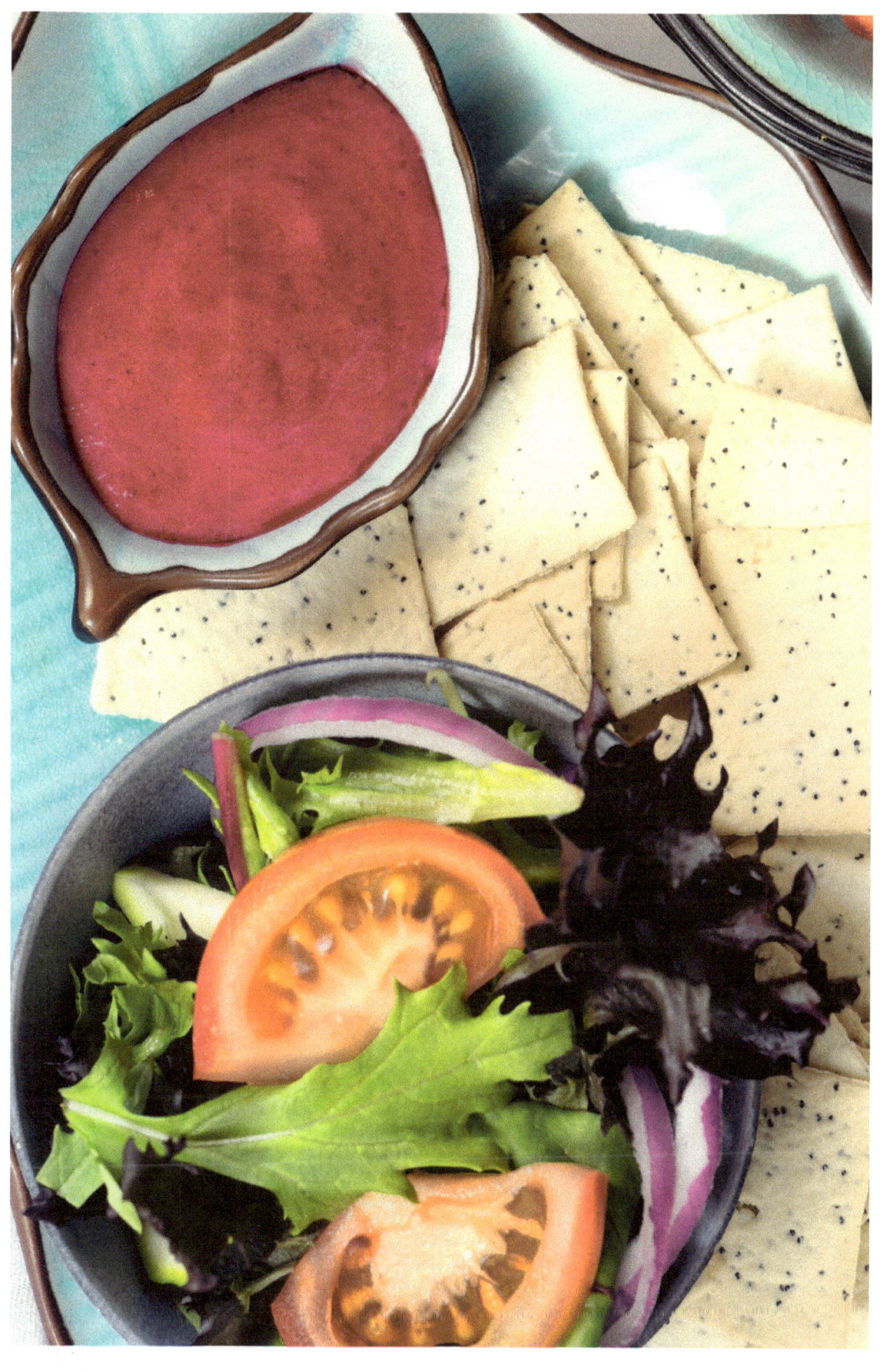

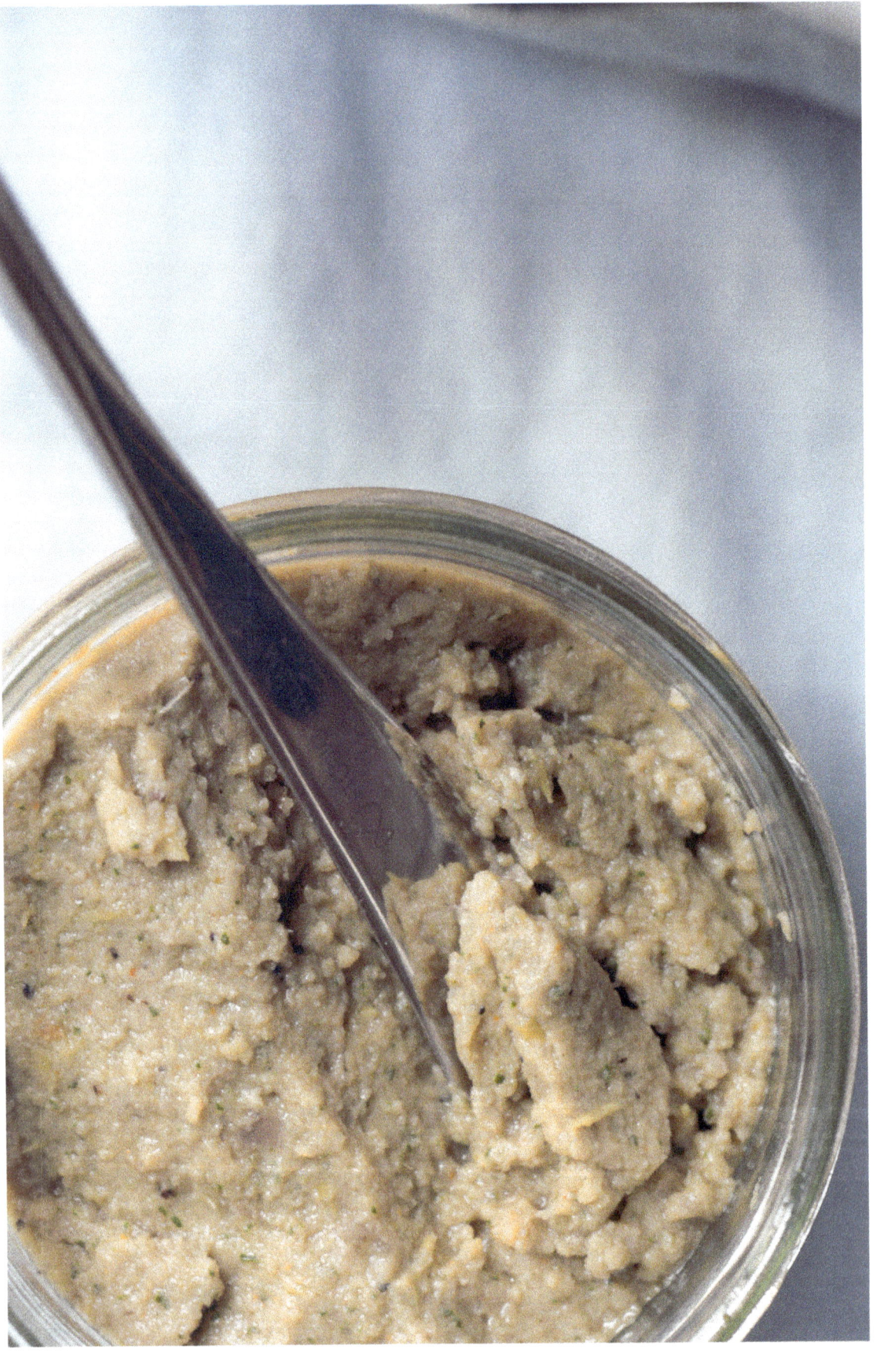

HOT GREEN PAPRIKA PÂTÉ

KCAL 37 | PROTEIN 2.6g | FAT 1.8g | CARBS 3.4g | SERVES 8

INGREDIENTS

1–2 green paprika peppers

1 red onion

3 cloves garlic

pinch of salt

1 tsp extra-virgin olive oil

300g soft tofu

1 tbsp lime juice

¼ cup soy milk

¼ cup fresh mint

1 tsp smoked paprika powder

METHOD

1. Wash and slice the paprika peppers and place on a baking tray. Peel and slice the red onion and garlic and place on the same tray. Sprinkle with salt and spray with the olive oil then bake at medium temperature for 15 minutes or until they start to turn golden. Remove from the oven and set aside to cool.

2. When cool, blend the roasted vegetables with the remaining ingredients, adding the soy milk incrementally until the desired consistency is achieved.

3. Transfer the pâté into a jam jar or serving dish and cover. Refrigerate to set. Keep in the refrigerator and consume within 3–5 days.

Notes

1. Green paprika peppers are available at Asian grocers. You can also use jalapeño peppers or capsicums, according to your preferred level of heat.

2. You can also add ¼ tsp cumin or coriander seeds.

3. You can achieve a firmer consistency using soft tofu, but silken tofu may also be used.

SPICY SALSA DIP

KCAL 44 | PROTEIN 2.6g | FAT 0.6g | CARBS 9g | SERVES 4

INGREDIENTS

2 spring onions

2 medium tomatoes

1 shallot

2 cloves garlic

1 tbsp lemon juice

pinch of salt

1 tbsp nutritional yeast flakes

1 tbsp coriander

2 red chilli peppers (see note)

For the garnish
Fresh coriander

METHOD

1. Wash the spring onions and tomatoes and finely chop. Peel and finely slice the shallot and crush the garlic.

2. Mix the vegetables in a bowl together with the lemon juice, salt and yeast flakes.

3. Wash and chop the coriander. Wash the chilli peppers and slice finely. Combine all the ingredients, setting aside some of the coriander for a garnish. Cover and set aside for 2–3 hours for the flavours to develop.

4. Garnish with remaining coriander and serve.

Note

1. You can substitute the red chilli peppers with ½ tsp cayenne pepper.

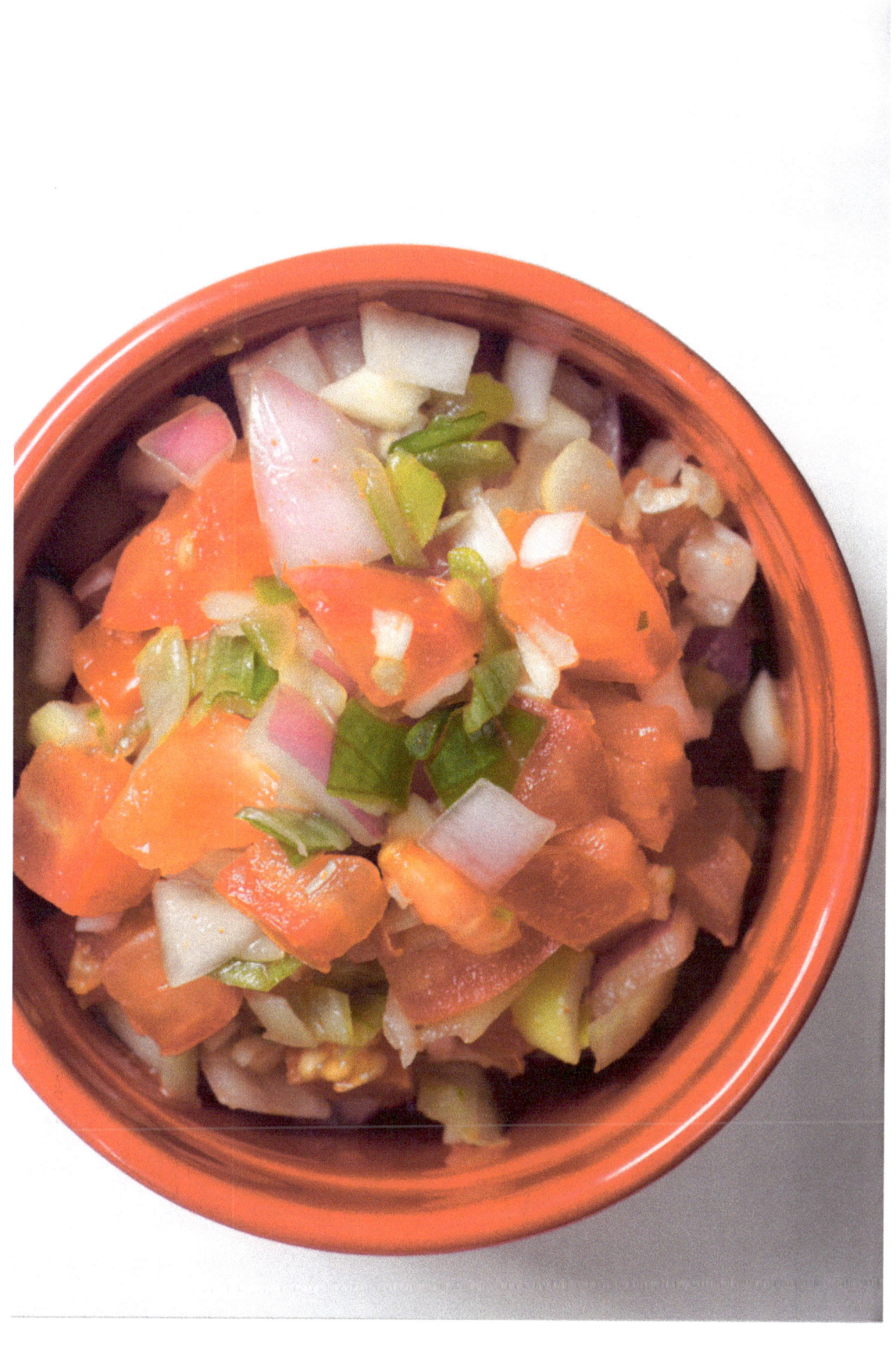

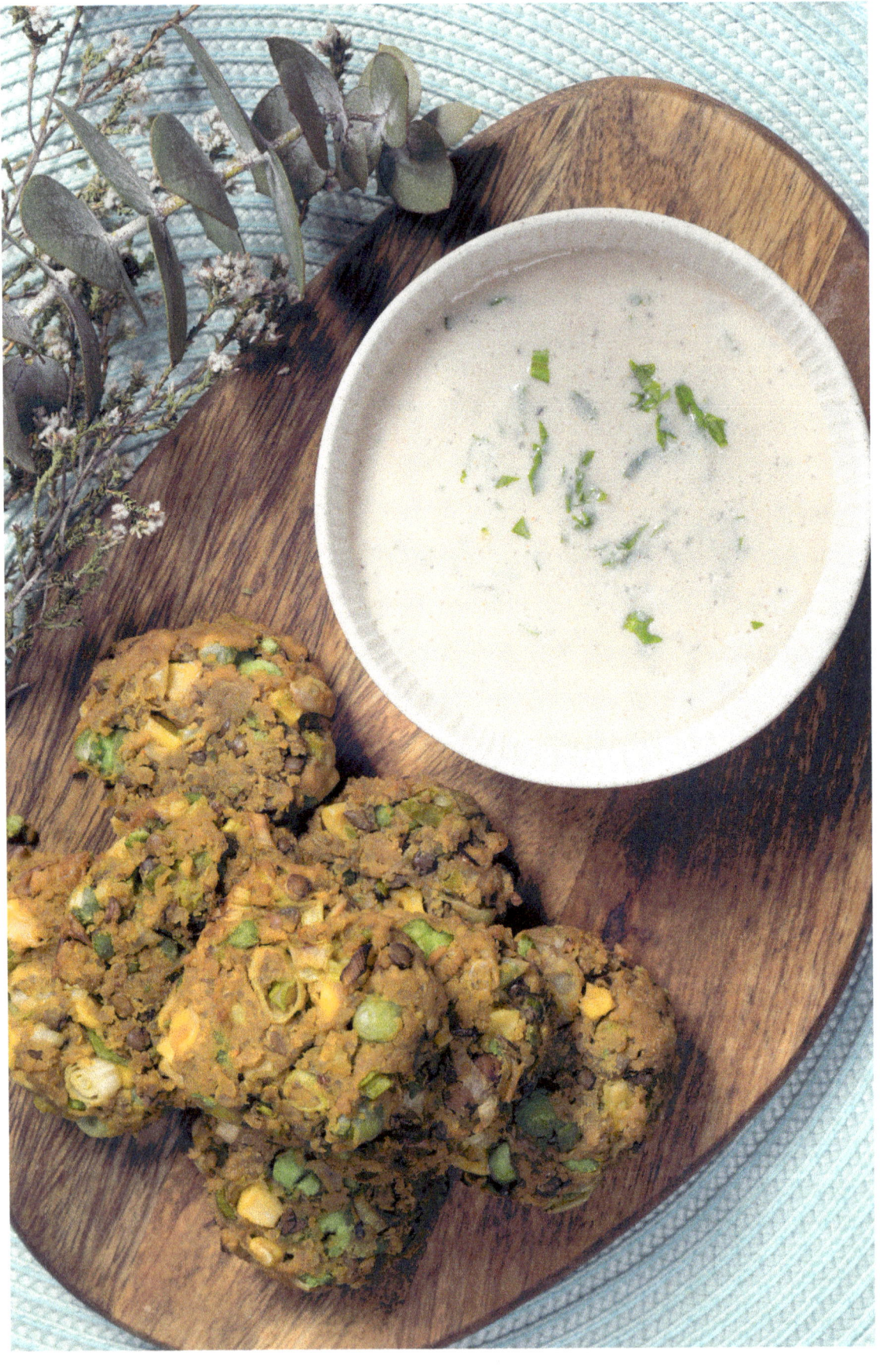

PEA & SWEETCORN NUGGETS WITH GARLIC AIOLI

KCAL 151 | PROTEIN 8.7g | FAT 6.3g | CARBS 17.8g | SERVES 10 (2 nuggets per serve)

INGREDIENTS

For the nuggets

½ cup TVP, finely ground

50g mixed lentils (brown, orange and urad dahl)

25g dried peas

25g bulgur wheat

2 cups vegetable stock

2 tbsp apple cider vinegar

1 leek, sliced

2 cloves garlic, crushed

pinch of salt and black pepper

3 spring onions, finely sliced

1 small zucchini, grated

2 carrots, grated

125g sweetcorn

4 tbsp nutritional yeast flakes

4 tbsp lentil flour

100g ground almonds

½ tsp turmeric

1 tsp each sage, rosemary and thyme

½ tsp onion powder

For the creamy garlic aioli

See recipe on page 52

METHOD

1. Pre-soak the TVP, mixed lentils and peas for at least 12 hours and thoroughly rinse several times with a sieve until the water runs clear.

2. Rinse and drain the bulgur wheat and place together with the TVP and lentils mix in a pan with the stock, apple cider vinegar, leek, garlic and seasoning.

3. Bring to the boil and simmer. Add additional water incrementally until the lentils are cooked and there is no excess liquid. Set aside to cool.

4. Meanwhile, combine the sliced spring onions, grated zucchini, grated carrots, sweetcorn, nutritional yeast flakes, lentil flour and ground almonds in another bowl.

5. Combine vegetable mixture with the cooled lentils mixture until well mixed. The consistency should be firm but not solid. If the mixture is too dry add some water to loosen it. If it is too runny add a little more lentil flour.

6. Roll the mixture into 20 small balls and press onto a non-stick baking tray to form nugget shapes. Bake on medium heat for 10–15 minutes or until golden brown, turning once.

7. Serve with creamy garlic aioli or a dip of your choice.

Notes

1. The nutritional information does not include the 'Creamy garlic aioli'.

2. 'Urad dahl' are also called 'split lentils' or 'black gram'.

CREAMY GARLIC AIOLI DIP

KCAL 36 | PROTEIN 2.5g | FAT 2.6g | CARBS 1.5g | SERVES 10

INGREDIENTS

3 cloves garlic

1 tbsp fresh basil, chopped

1 tbsp fresh oregano, chopped

300g silken tofu

3 tbsp light soy milk

½ tsp paprika powder

½ tsp cayenne pepper

1 tbsp apple cider vinegar

pinch of black salt

pinch of black pepper

1 tsp mustard

METHOD

1. Peel the garlic. Rinse and drain the tofu.

2. Combine all the ingredients except the herbs in a blender and blend until smooth.

3. Stir in the herbs with a sprinkle on top to serve.

Notes

1. You can use soft tofu in place of the silken tofu for a firmer consistency.

2. You can adjust the consistency by adding more or less soy milk.

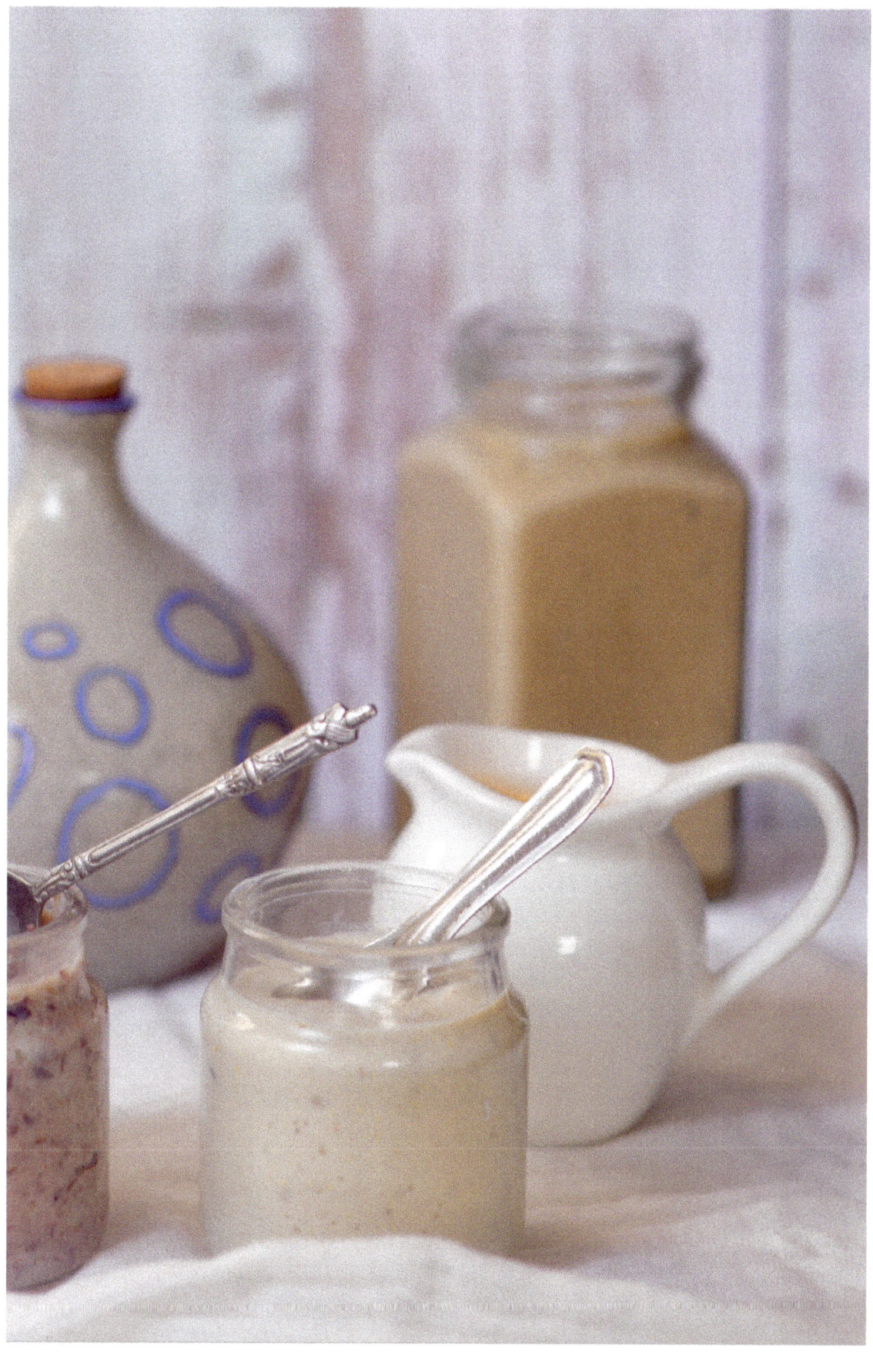

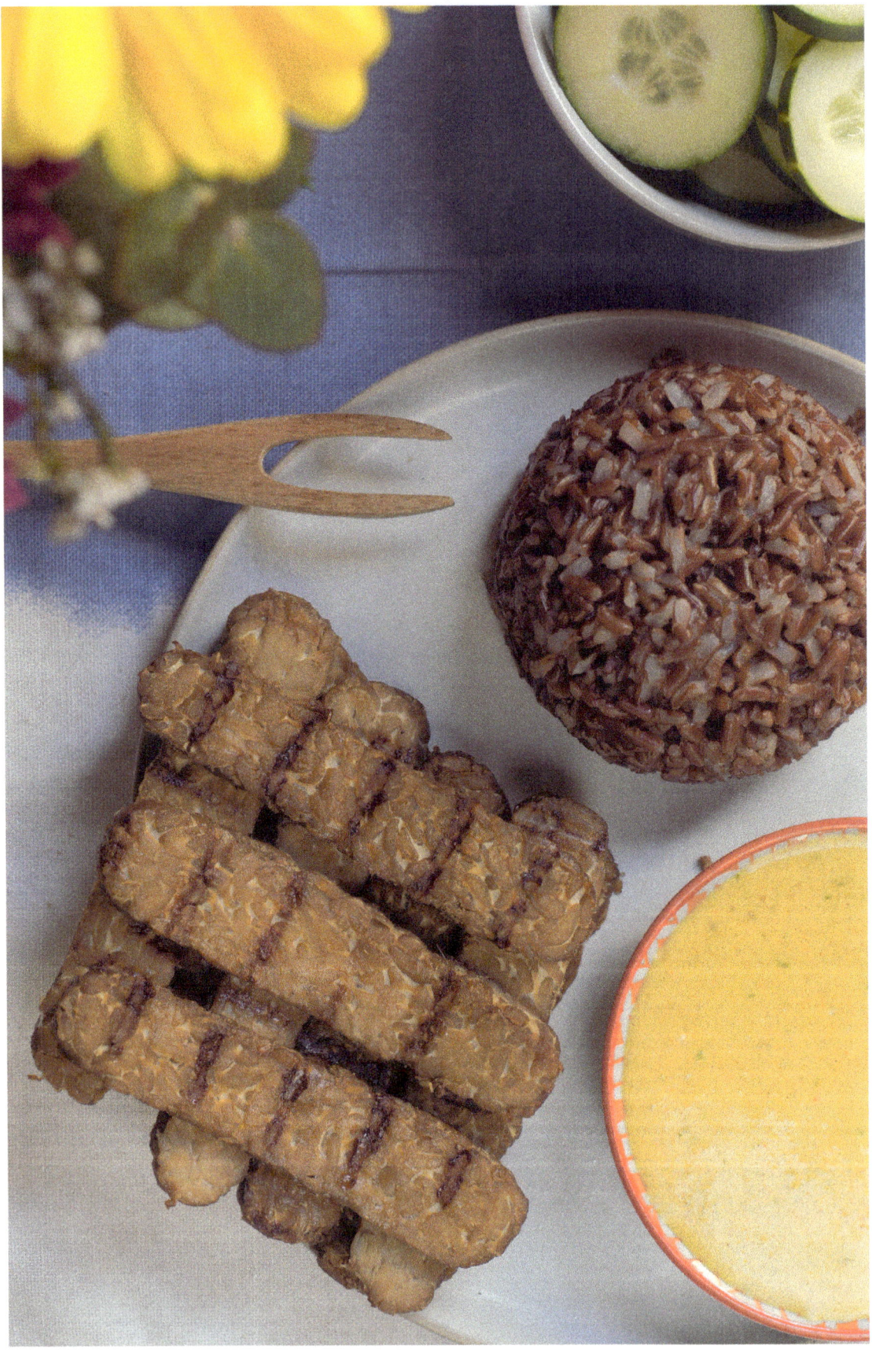

MAINS

Explore a range of possibilities to create incredibly tasty and varied high-protein dishes entirely from plant food sources.

This collection of mains include whole grains, seeds, legumes and textured vegetable protein, but it's tofu and tempeh that steal the show! They boast high-protein content as well as being sources of omega-3, vitamins, minerals, antioxidants and other healthy plant-based compounds. Tempeh has a slightly lower protein content, and as a fermented food, it complements tofu with prebiotics and other plant-based compounds. We love using both tofu and tempeh in our dishes.

'Firm' or 'extra-firm' tofu are the types of tofu most commonly used in these recipes. For tempeh, we use 'unmarinated', 'fresh', 'frozen' or 'raw' tempeh, that has not been marinated.

These recipes contain a variety of plant-based protein sources. If you would like to use seitan, which is a protein-rich food extracted from wheat, feel free to substitute in place of tofu or tempeh.

A variety of cooking styles have been used, including steaming in *'Peanut and sweet potato tofu stack'*, and grilling or barbecuing for *'Tofu skewers'* and baking in *'Lemon-glazed tofu steak'*.

Some recipes are super-easy to make, such as *'Easy cheesy pasta'*, and some require more preparation, such as *'Tempeh tomato stacks'*. Whichever is right for you, we hope you have fun trying them out, experimenting with your ingredients – and make these recipes your own!

TANTALISING TORTILLAS

KCAL 349 | PROTEIN 20g | FAT 15g | CARBS 42g | SERVES 2 (2 tortillas per serve)

INGREDIENTS

4 corn tortillas

4 tbsp black beans, cooked

pinch of salt

handful of rocket leaves

For the tofu

200g firm tofu

pinch of black salt and black pepper or to taste

¼ tsp turmeric

1 tbsp nutritional yeast flakes

For the guacamole

3 green onions

1 red chilli pepper

1 medium tomato

½ avocado

2 cloves garlic, crushed

1 tbsp lemon juice

pinch of salt

For the salsa

4 large tbsp salsa (see recipe page 48)

METHOD

1. **For the tofu** – Rinse, drain and crumble tofu into a bowl. Mix in the salt (black salt is best), pepper, turmeric and yeast flakes.

2. **For the black beans** – Rinse and drain well. Sprinkle with salt and set aside.

3. **For the guacamole** – Wash and finely chop the green onions, chilli pepper and tomato. In a bowl mash the avocado and combine with the tomato mixture and add the remaining guacamole ingredients. Season with salt to taste.

4. **Make up the tortillas** – Warm each tortilla in a sandwich press or grill on one side. Then flip over and warm the opposite side. Add a helping of tofu, sprinkle with black beans, stuff in some rocket and cover with salsa. Fold in half and cook in a sandwich press or grill until tortilla begins to brown. Add guacamole to each one or serve as a side.

Notes

1. The nutritional information does not include the *'Spicy salsa dip'*.

2. Tortillas can be home-made or store purchased.

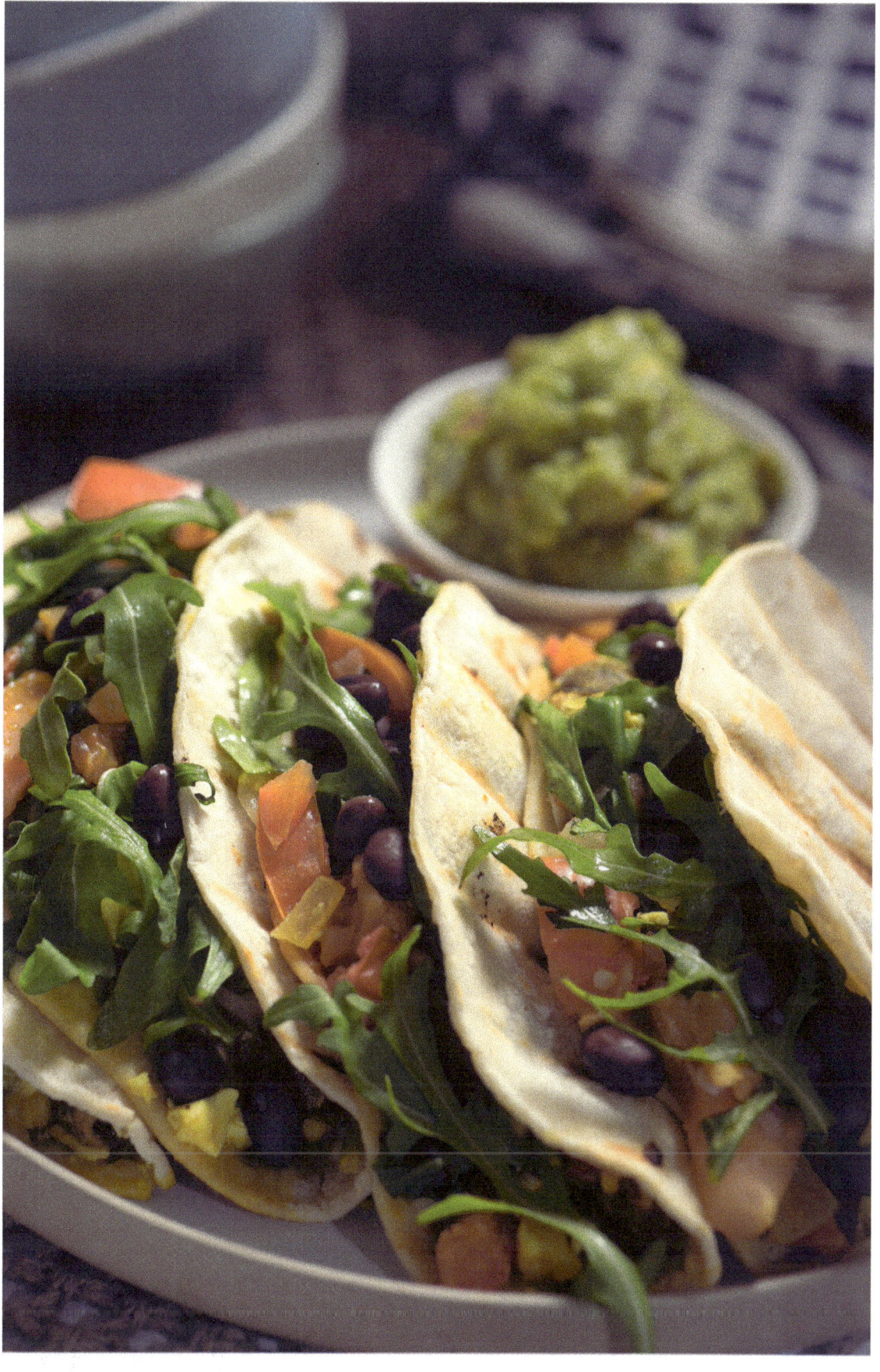

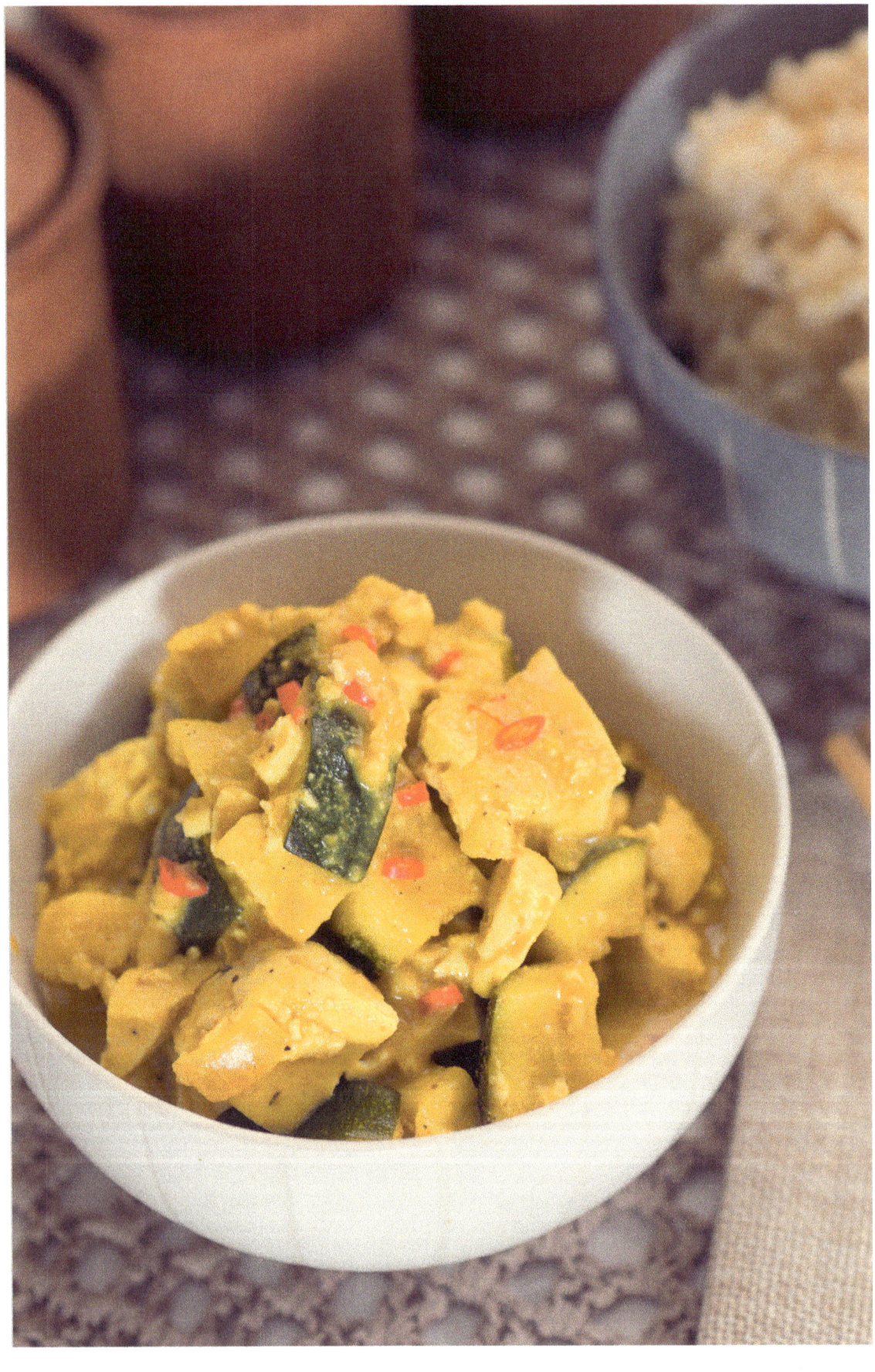

YELLOW TOFU CURRY

KCAL 234 | PROTEIN 21g | FAT 9.8g | CARBS 22g | SERVES 4

INGREDIENTS

500g firm tofu

2 cloves garlic, crushed

2 shallots, finely chopped

1 tsp extra-virgin olive oil

½ tsp turmeric

½ tsp cayenne pepper or to taste

¼ tsp cumin powder

½ tsp nutmeg

pinch of salt

pinch of black pepper

1 stick lemongrass, chopped (optional)

1 stick ginger, peeled and grated

2 cups mixed seasonal vegetables, chopped

2 tbsp lemon juice

2 tbsp light soy sauce

4 tbsp nutritional yeast flakes

1 cup light soy milk

For the garnish

2 tsp fresh coriander, chopped

METHOD

1. Rinse and drain the tofu. Cut into cubes and pat dry.

2. Sauté the garlic and shallots in the olive oil then add the tofu cubes and spices (turmeric, cayenne pepper, cumin powder, nutmeg, salt and pepper). Add the chopped lemongrass (if using) and grated ginger and cook for a further 30 seconds.

3. Add the mixed seasonal vegetables, lemon juice, soy sauce, nutritional yeast and soy milk. Cook on low heat until vegetables are just soft.

4. Serve garnished with chopped coriander.

Notes

1. Choose veggies that are in season near you. Veggies that work well in this dish are carrot, zucchini, tomato, baby sweetcorn, snap peas, mushroom, cauliflower and eggplant – grill the eggplant first by cutting into slices then sprinkle with salt on a non-stick grill.

2. If you don't have fresh ginger, substitute with ½ tsp ginger powder.

MUSHROOM PENNE

KCAL 292 | PROTEIN 15g | FAT 6.9g | CARBS 44g | SERVES 4

INGREDIENTS

1 cup dried shiitake mushrooms

1 cup water

2 cloves garlic

1½ cups penne pasta

2 shallots, finely chopped

1 tbsp extra-virgin olive oil

pinch of salt

pinch of black pepper

2 tsp cornflour

2 cups light soy milk

1 tbsp light soy sauce

1 tbsp malt extract

6 tbsp nutritional yeast flakes

METHOD

1. Pre-soak the dried mushrooms in the water overnight, retaining the water as mushroom stock. Wash and slice the mushrooms and crush the garlic.

2. Bring a pan of salted water to the boil and add the penne pasta. Cook until 'al dente' tender.

3. Sauté the garlic and shallots in the olive oil with salt and pepper.

4. Mix the cornflour into 2 tbsp of the soy milk with a fork until it is smooth and without lumps. Add this back into the remaining soy milk.

5. Add the mushrooms with the mushroom stock, the soy milk mixed with the cornflour, light soy sauce, malt extract and nutritional yeast flakes to the pan. Keep on medium heat, stirring until the mushrooms are cooked and the sauce has thickened.

6. Portion the pasta onto serving plates and spoon the mushroom sauce on top.

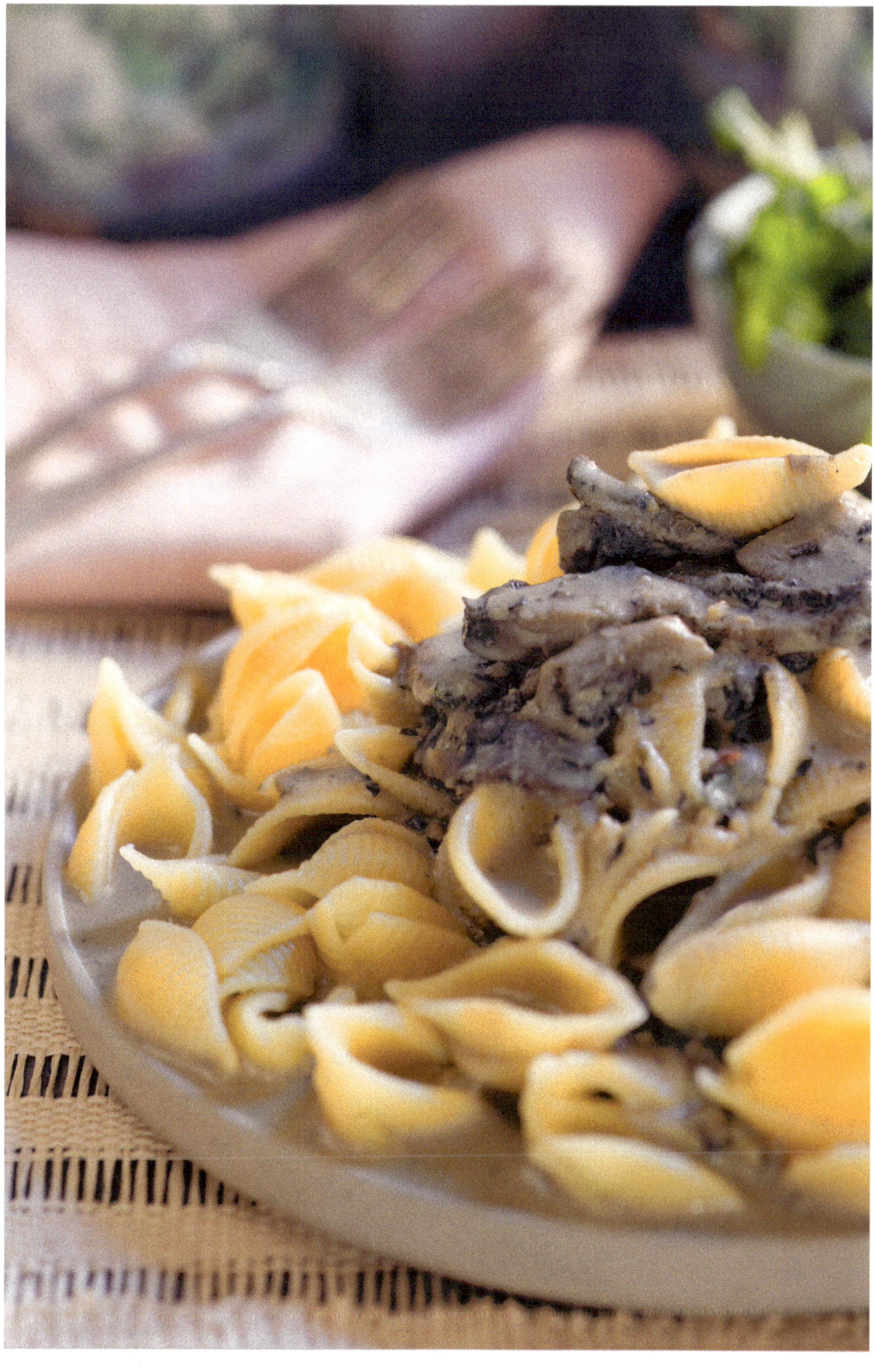

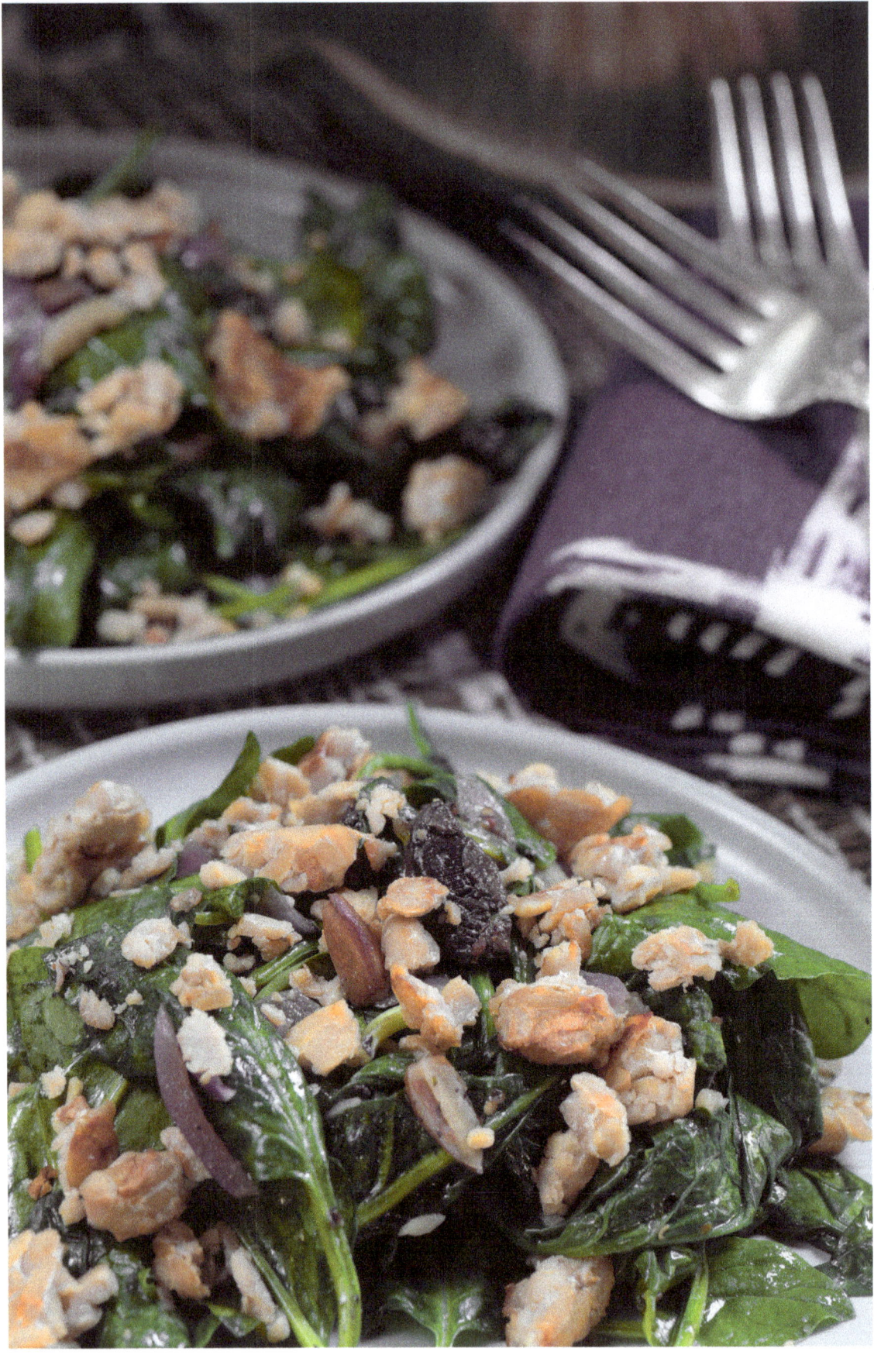

TEMPEH MEDLEY

KCAL 203 | PROTEIN 14g | FAT 13g | CARBS 13g | SERVES 4

INGREDIENTS

8 cups fresh spinach

1 red onion

¼ cup almonds

2 dried apricots

200g tempeh

1 tbsp extra-virgin olive oil

1 tsp Dijon mustard

1 tbsp vinegar

pinch of salt

pinch of black pepper

½ tsp cayenne pepper

METHOD

1. Wash the spinach thoroughly, drain and chop. Peel and thinly slice the onion, slice the almonds and chop the apricots. Set aside.

2. Slice the tempeh and grill evenly on both sides. Set aside.

3. Sauté the onion and almonds in the olive oil and add the mustard, vinegar, salt, black pepper and cayenne pepper.

4. Turn off the heat and combine the spinach into the pan.

5. Crumble the grilled tempeh into smaller pieces and add to the mixture with the apricots.

6. Serve.

SPINACH RISONI

KCAL 329 | PROTEIN 17g | FAT 8.8g | CARBS 46g | SERVES 4

INGREDIENTS

4 cups spinach

1 onion

2 cloves garlic

1 tbsp extra-virgin olive oil

pinch of salt

pinch of black pepper

1½ cups risoni pasta

4 cups light soy milk

½ tsp nutmeg

1 tbsp malt extract

For the garnish

2 tsp fresh parsley, chopped

METHOD

1. Wash the spinach thoroughly, drain and chop. Peel and chop the onion and garlic.

2. Sauté the onion and garlic in a pan with the olive oil, salt and pepper.

3. Add the pasta and soy milk to the pan and simmer for 15 minutes or until pasta is cooked.

4. Add the nutmeg, malt extract and spinach, combine well and simmer for 30 seconds.

5. Serve with fresh chopped parsley to garnish.

Note

1. You can substitute risoni pasta with orzo pasta.

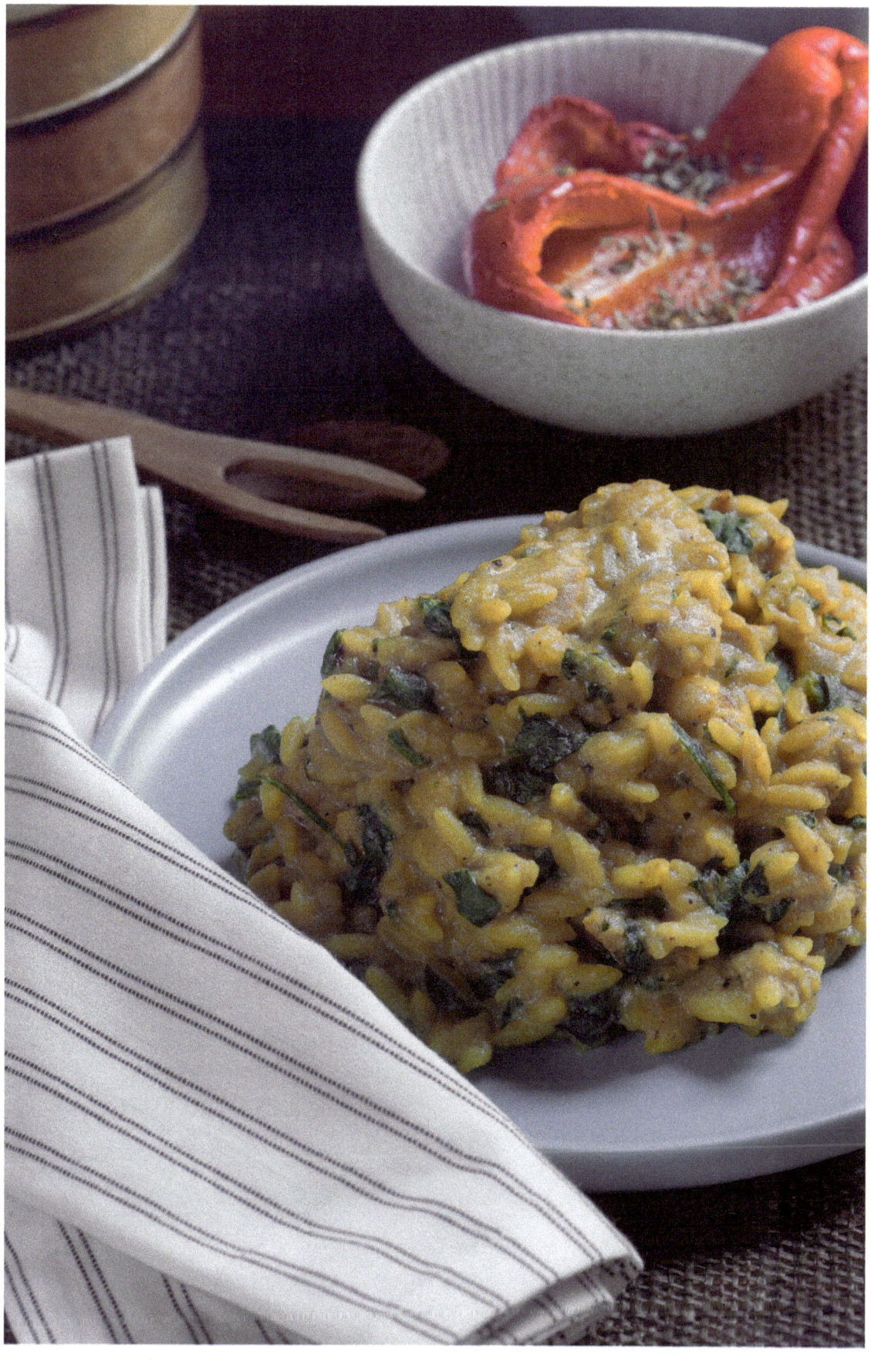

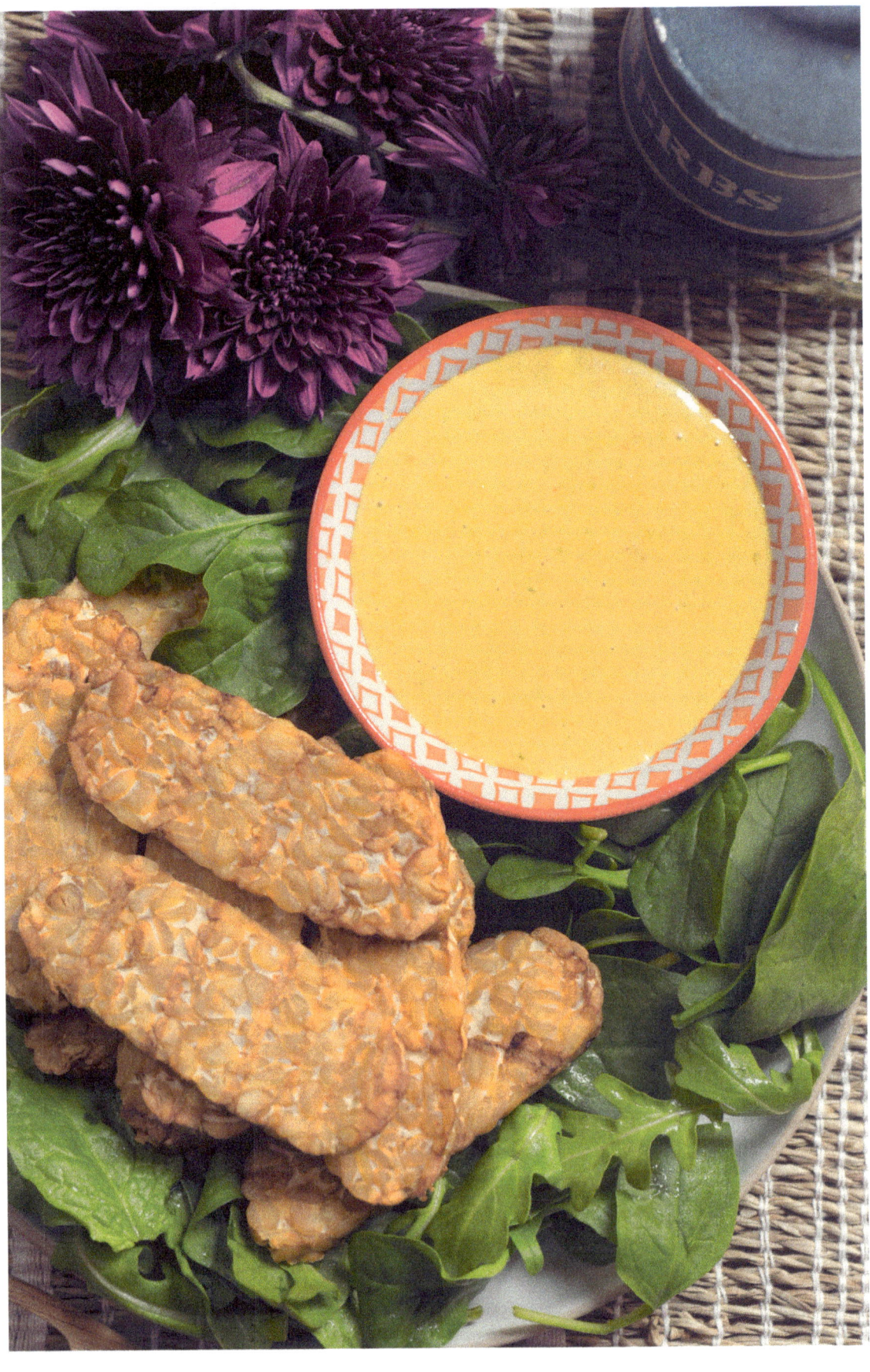

TEMPEH SATAY

KCAL 343 | PROTEIN 21g | FAT 20g | CARBS 25g | SERVES 6

INGREDIENTS

500g tempeh

For the satay sauce

75g peanuts

5 spring onions

pinch of salt

½ tsp cumin powder

½ tsp turmeric powder

½ tsp ginger powder

1 stick lemongrass

2 cloves garlic

75ml thick coconut cream (unsweetened)

200ml water

1 tsp tamarind extract

1 tsp cayenne pepper

1 tbsp apple cider vinegar

20g candlenuts (optional)

2 fresh chilli peppers

METHOD

1. Toast the peanuts by arranging them on a baking tray and slow-toasting on a low heat. Be sure to watch them as they can burn very quickly. Remove from heat when done and set aside.

2. Slice the tempeh and grill evenly on both sides.

3. Meanwhile prepare the satay sauce by combining the toasted peanuts with remaining ingredients in a blender.

4. Serve the tempeh and satay sauce with a salad.

Notes

1. The satay sauce will keep for 3 days in the fridge.

2. Tamarind extract can be substituted with mango powder, or 2 tbsp lemon juice.

3. Fresh chilli peppers can be substituted with chilli flakes.

CAPSICUM ROASTED TOFU

KCAL 207 | PROTEIN 18g | FAT 11g | CARBS 15g | SERVES 2

INGREDIENTS

300g extra-firm tofu

2 capsicums (bell peppers), cubed

2 tomatoes, cubed

2 red chilli peppers, sliced (optional)

For the marinade

1 tbsp light soy sauce

1 tbsp sweet soy sauce

2 cloves garlic, crushed

1-inch stick ginger, peeled and grated

½ tsp cumin powder

1 tsp extra-virgin olive oil

1 tbsp vegan fish sauce (optional)

For the garnish

Fresh coriander

METHOD

1. **For the marinade** – Combine light soy sauce, sweet soy sauce, garlic, ginger, cumin powder, olive oil and vegan fish sauce (if using).

2. **For the tofu** – Rinse and drain the tofu and cut into cubes. Place into a dish with the marinade. Let it sit for 6 hours or overnight in the fridge.

3. Take the marinated tofu and place with the marinade into a baking dish. Add the cubed tomato, capsicum and chilli peppers (if using) and stir carefully to combine. Check seasoning and adjust if necessary.

4. Bake using medium heat for 20 minutes or until tofu starts to turn golden brown.

5. Serve garnished with fresh coriander.

Note

1. Fresh red chilli peppers can be substituted with chilli flakes or black pepper according to your taste.

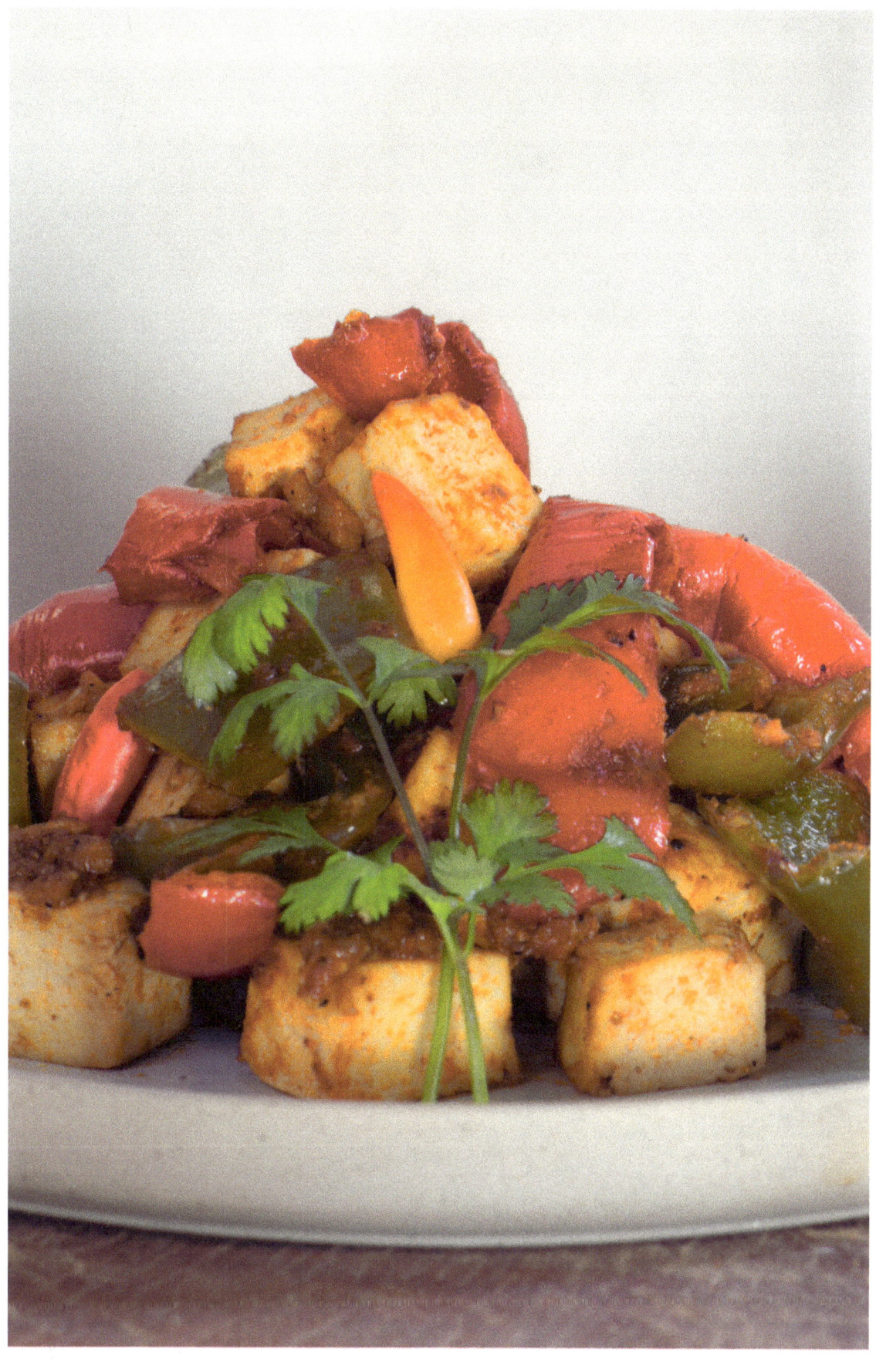

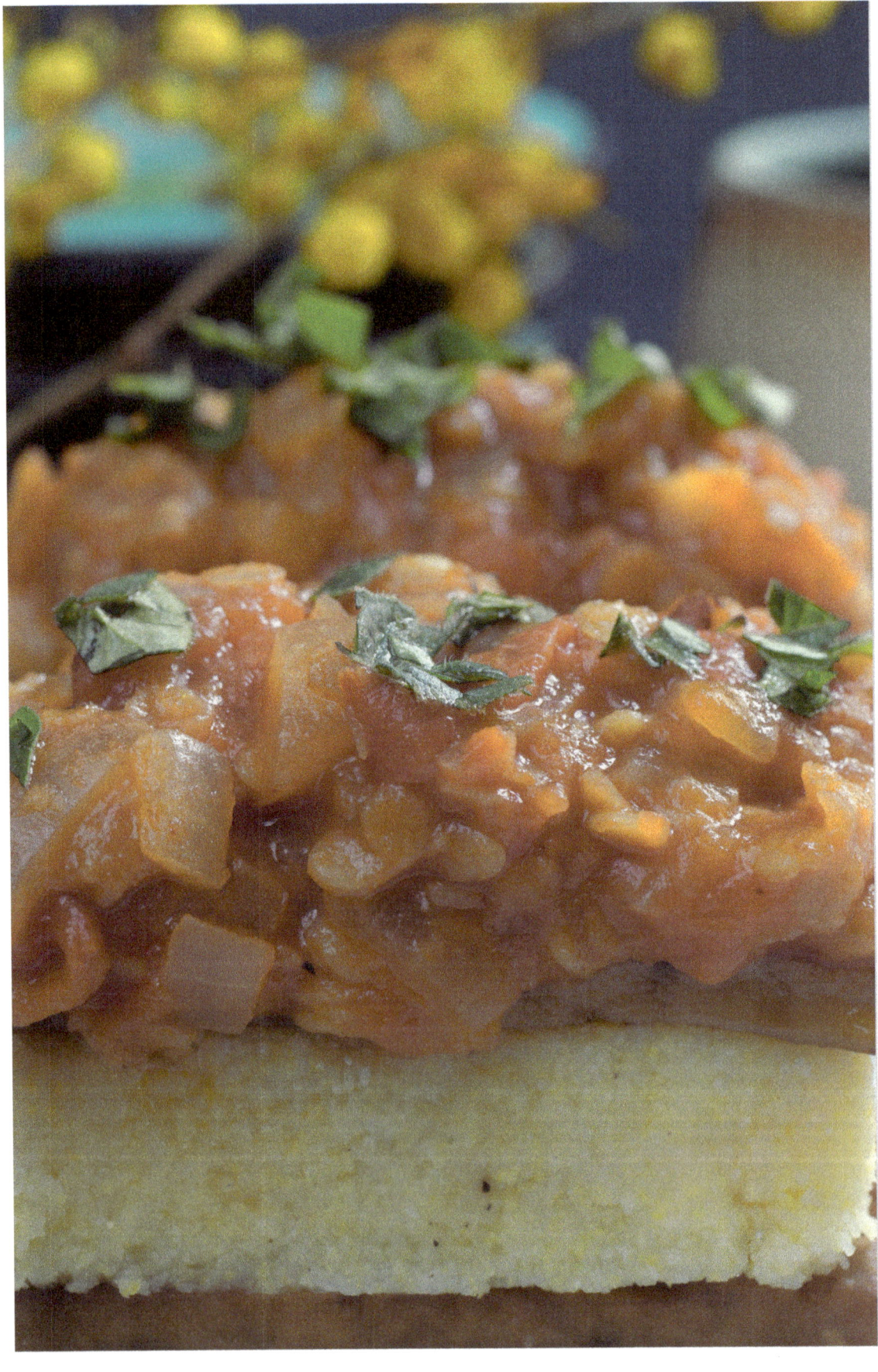

TEMPEH TOMATO STACKS

KCAL 313 | PROTEIN 24g | FAT 14g | CARBS 26g | SERVES 6 (2 stacks per serve)

INGREDIENTS

500g tempeh

For the polenta

1 cup polenta

1¾ cups light soy milk

pinch of salt or to taste

pinch of black pepper

For the tomato sauce

1 onion

2 cloves garlic

1 tbsp extra-virgin olive oil

½ cup orange lentils

2 tbsp lemon juice

1 fresh red chilli pepper, chopped

2 tbsp tomato paste

1½ cups water

pinch of salt or to taste

pinch of black pepper

For the garnish

Fresh oregano, chopped

METHOD

1. **For the tempeh** – Cut the tempeh blocks into 12 slices each. Grill evenly on both sides.

2. **For the polenta** – Place the polenta in a pan and cover with 1 cup light soy milk and add salt and pepper to taste. Bring to the boil and cook on low heat for 2–3 minutes. Set aside.

3. **For the tomato sauce** – Peel and chop the onion and garlic. Sauté the onion and garlic in the olive oil until they begin to change colour.

4. Rinse and drain the lentils. Add the lentils with the remaining ingredients for the tomato sauce, bring to boil and simmer for 10–15 minutes or until lentils are soft. Add more water if necessary.

5. **To build the stacks** – Start with a layer of tempeh on the bottom, polenta sandwiched in the middle, and a topping of the tomato lentil mixture. Make 12 stacks in total – each stack has 2 slices of tempeh. Garnish with fresh chopped oregano and enjoy.

Notes

1. Fresh red chilli peppers can be substituted with chilli powder.

EASY CHEESY PASTA

KCAL 374 | PROTEIN 22g | FAT 7.7g | CARBS 54g | SERVES 4

INGREDIENTS

2 cups pasta

For the cheesy sauce

2 tsp cornflour

4 cups light soy milk

2 cloves garlic, crushed

6 tbsp nutritional yeast flakes

2 tbsp apple cider vinegar

1 tsp Italian herbs

pinch of salt

pinch of black pepper

For the garnish

2 tsp oregano, chopped

METHOD

1. Bring a pan of salted water to the boil and add the pasta. Simmer for 10-15 minutes or until pasta is cooked 'al dente'. Drain and set aside.

2. **For the sauce** – Combine the cornflour with the soy milk, garlic, nutritional yeast and apple cider vinegar in a blender. Blend until smooth.

3. Place the sauce in a pan with the Italian herbs and seasoning and cook on a medium heat, stirring, for 10–15 minutes or until sauce thickens.

4. Serve the sauce over the pasta with oregano garnish.

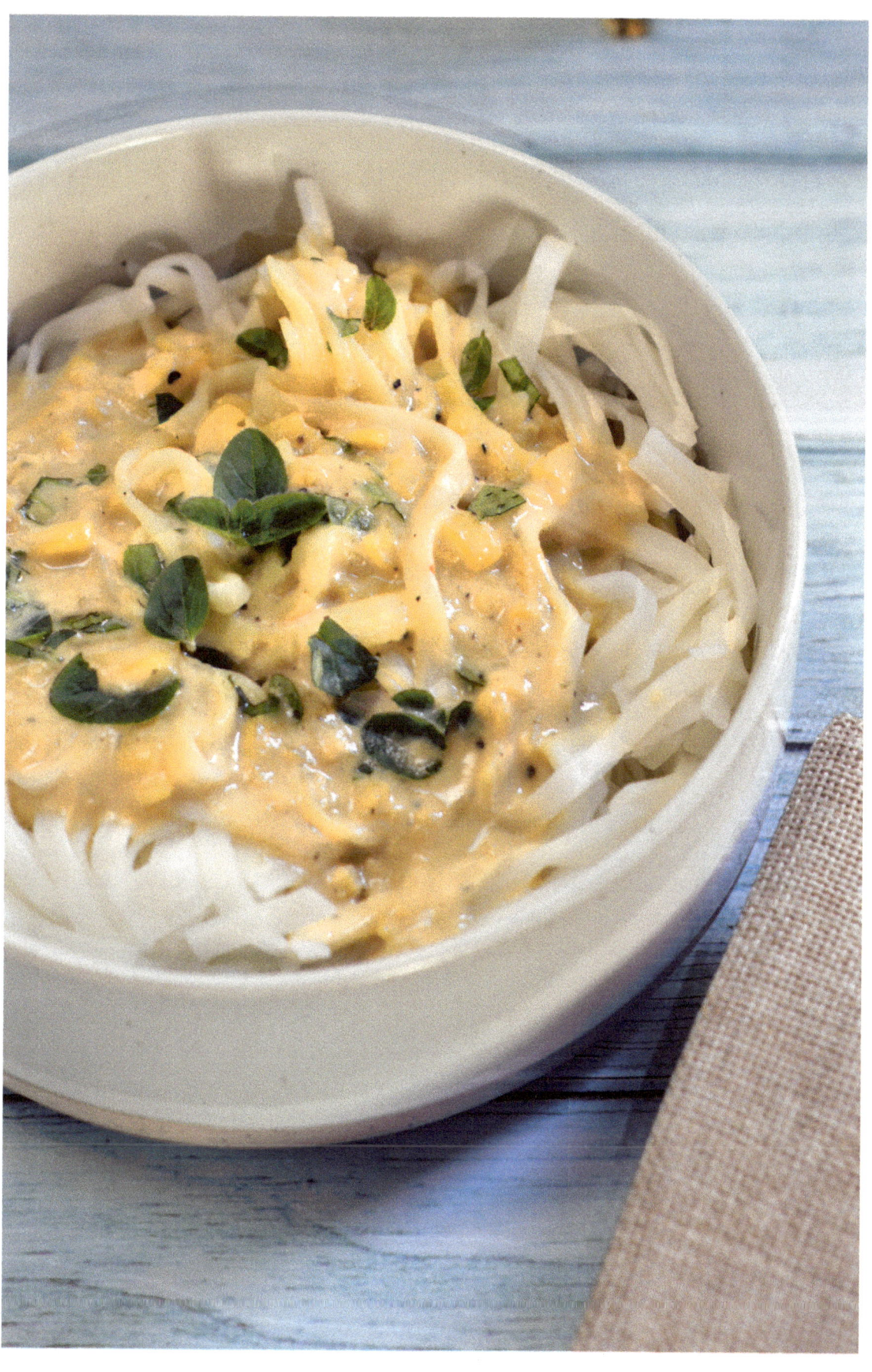

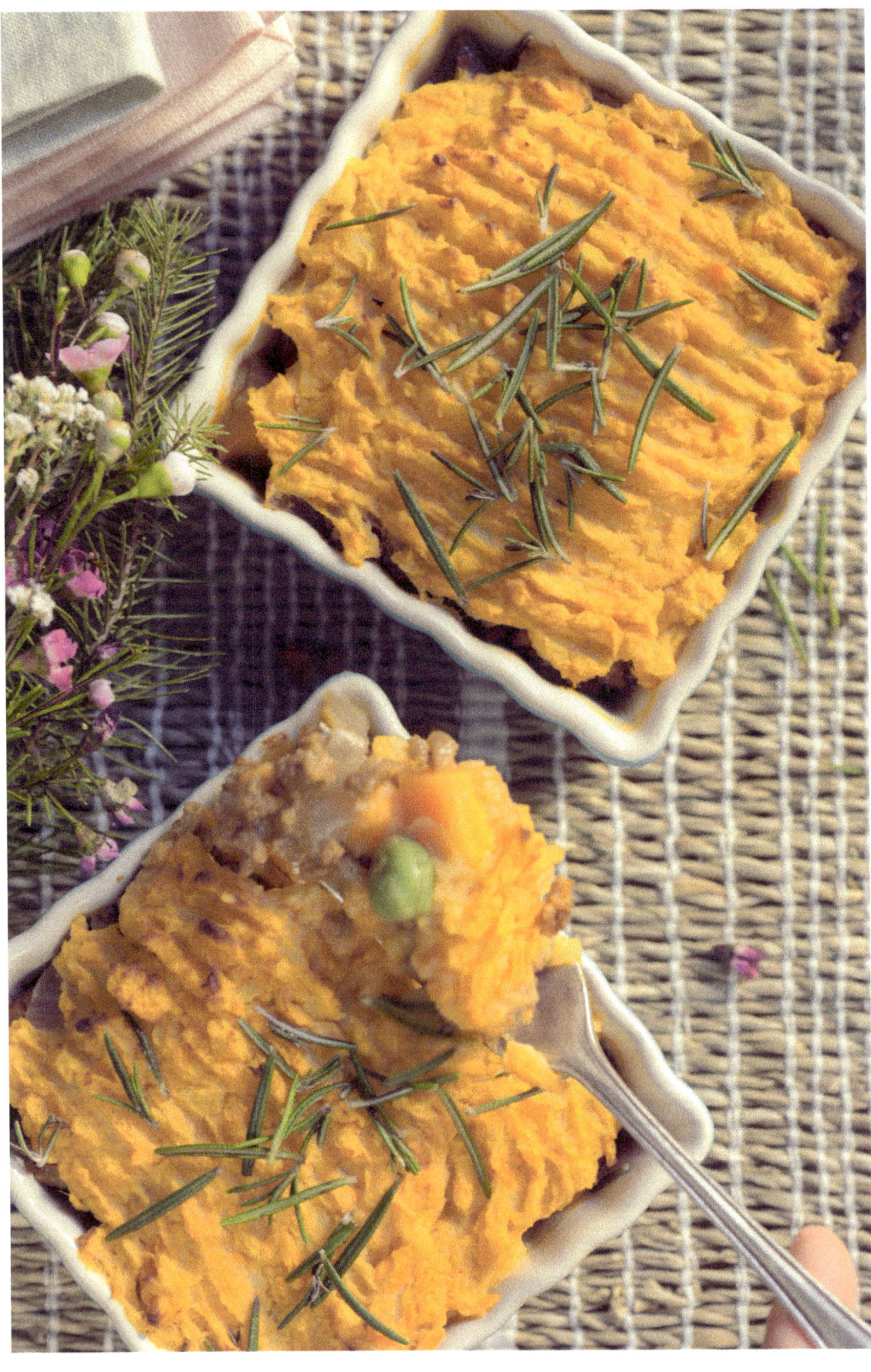

NO MEAT SHEPHERD'S PIE

KCAL 284 | PROTEIN 15g | FAT 6.3g | CARBS 45g | SERVES 6

INGREDIENTS

¾ cup TVP (see note)

¼ cup mixed orange lentils and quinoa

2 onions

1 leek

2 tomatoes

2 carrots

2 sticks celery

2 cloves garlic, crushed

2 tbsp extra-virgin olive oil

pinch of salt and black pepper

50g fresh peas

2 tbsp malt extract

1 tbsp soy sauce

2 tbsp apple cider vinegar

2 tbsp tomato paste

1–2 tbsp fresh rosemary

½ tsp thyme

4 bay leaves

For the topping

3 medium sweet potatoes

¼ cup light soy milk

4 tbsp nutritional yeast flakes

pinch of salt and black pepper to taste

METHOD

1. Soak the TVP, lentils and quinoa in salted water overnight. Rinse thoroughly until the water runs clear and drain.

2. Finely chop the onions, leek, tomatoes, carrots and celery. Roughly chop the sweet potatoes.

3. Prepare the mash by boiling the sweet potatoes in salted water until soft. Drain and set the cooking water aside as vegetable stock.

4. Sauté the onions, leek and garlic in the oil with the salt and pepper. Add the TVP, lentils, quinoa, tomatoes, carrots, celery, peas, malt extract, soy sauce, apple cider vinegar, tomato paste and herbs with ¾ cup of the vegetable stock and bring to the boil. Simmer for 5–6 minutes.

5. Place the TVP mixture in an oven-proof dish.

6. Mash the sweet potatoes and stir in the soy milk, yeast flakes and salt and pepper to taste. Spoon the mash over the TVP.

7. Bake for 10-15 minutes on medium or until browned.

Notes

1. If you don't have TVP, you can substitute with ½ cup green lentils soaked overnight (this will change the nutritional profile).

2. Orange lentils are also known as 'red lentils', 'split lentils' or 'masoor dahl'.

3. Fresh peas can be substituted with frozen peas.

TEMPEH CURRY

KCAL 368 | PROTEIN 20g | FAT 16g | CARBS 41g | SERVES 5

INGREDIENTS

400g tempeh

2 medium white potatoes

2–3 red chilli peppers

2 shallots

2 cloves garlic

1-inch stick ginger

1 stick lemongrass

1-inch stick fresh turmeric (optional)

1-inch stick galangal (optional)

10g candlenuts (about 3 nuts)

½ tsp coriander seeds

½ tsp nutmeg

1 tbsp olive oil

pinch of salt

pinch of black pepper

2 cups vegetable stock

5 tbsp coconut cream

For the garnish

fresh coriander, chopped

METHOD

1. Cut the tempeh into small rectangles and grill evenly on both sides. Set aside.

2. Peel and chop the potatoes and wash and chop the chilli peppers and set aside.

3. Peel the shallots, garlic, ginger and lemongrass and the turmeric and galagal if using. Place them with the candlenuts, coriander seeds, nutmeg and chilli peppers in a blender. Blend until fine. Sauté the blended mixture in the olive oil until it starts to change colour. Add the potatoes, salt and pepper and cook for approximately 1–2 minutes.

4. Add the vegetable stock and bring to the boil for 10 minutes. Add the tempeh and coconut cream and simmer for 2–3 minutes longer or until the potatoes are cooked.

5. Serve with a fresh coriander garnish.

Note

1. Fresh turmeric can be substituted with ½ tsp turmeric powder.

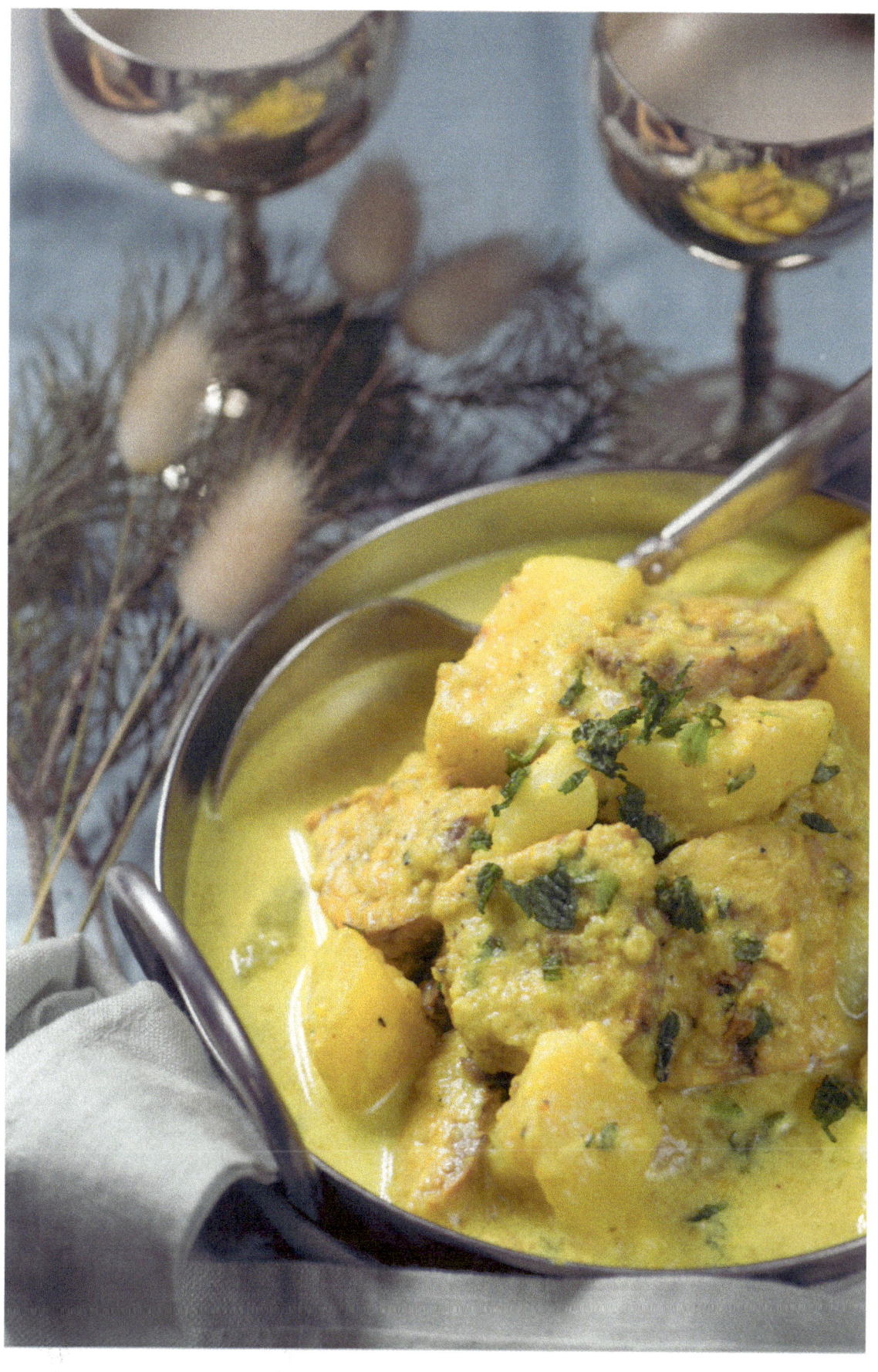

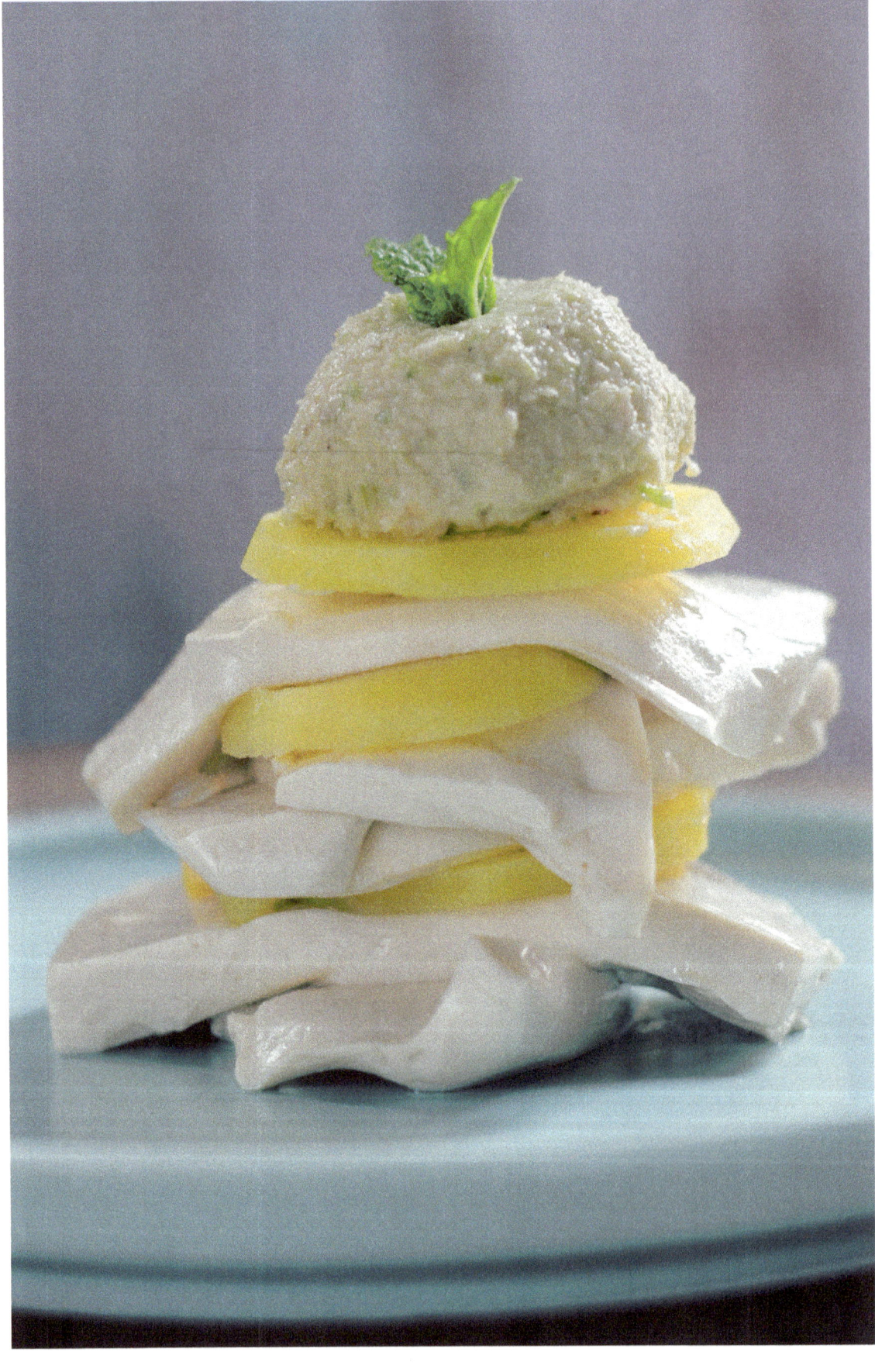

PEANUT & SWEET POTATO TOFU STACK

KCAL 306 | PROTEIN 20g | FAT 19g | CARBS 20g | SERVES 4

INGREDIENTS

500g semi-firm tofu

1 large sweet potato

pinch of salt

For the peanut chutney

100g roasted peanuts

2 spring onions

pinch of salt

2 tbsp lime juice

1-inch stick ginger, peeled

2 cloves garlic

5 tbsp water

1 tsp tamarind extract

1 fresh red chilli pepper

1 stick lemongrass, chopped

For the garnish

fresh mint leaves

METHOD

1. Rinse and drain the tofu and cut into slices. Peel the sweet potato and cut into slices. Place them in a steamer, sprinkle with salt and steam for about 10 minutes or until sweet potato is tender. Set aside to cool.

2. Toast the peanuts by arranging them on a baking tray and toasting for 5–10 minutes or until they start to turn golden. Be sure to watch them carefully as they burn quickly.

3. Combine the toasted peanuts with remaining chutney ingredients and blend. Adjust seasoning to taste.

4. Construct stacks with chutney on top and garnish with mint to serve.

Notes

1. Red chilli pepper can be substituted with chilli powder.

2. Tamarind can be substituted with ½ tsp mango powder or 1 tbsp lime juice.

MILLET PILAF

KCAL 333 | PROTEIN 18g | FAT 14g | CARBS 39g | SERVES 4

INGREDIENTS

1 cup millet

450g firm tofu

2 brown onions, chopped

1 tbsp extra-virgin olive oil

pinch of salt

¼ tsp turmeric

5 cardamom pods, crushed

2 star anise pods

3 cups vegetable stock

1 bulb fennel, chopped

2 carrots, finely chopped

2 sticks celery, chopped

150g sweetcorn kernels

100g fresh spinach

For the garnish

20 toasted almonds, sliced

1 tbsp fresh mint, chopped

1 tbsp fresh parsley, chopped

For the marinade

'Garlic and ginger marinade' **(see recipe on page 107)**

METHOD

1. Pre-soak the millet overnight, drain and rinse.

2. Rinse, drain and marinate the tofu for 2–3 hours or overnight using a marinade – we suggest *'Garlic and ginger marinade'* on page 107.

3. Sauté the onions in the oil with the salt, turmeric and millet until the millet starts to brown or give a nutty aroma.

4. Crush the cardamom pods and star anise in a spice bag and add to millet with the tofu and marinade, vegetable stock, chopped vegetables and sweetcorn. Simmer for 30 minutes, covered, or until the water is absorbed.

5. Stir in the spinach and stand, covered, for 2 minutes.

6. Fluff the millet and serve topped with almonds, mint and parsley.

Note

1. The nutritional information does not include the marinade.

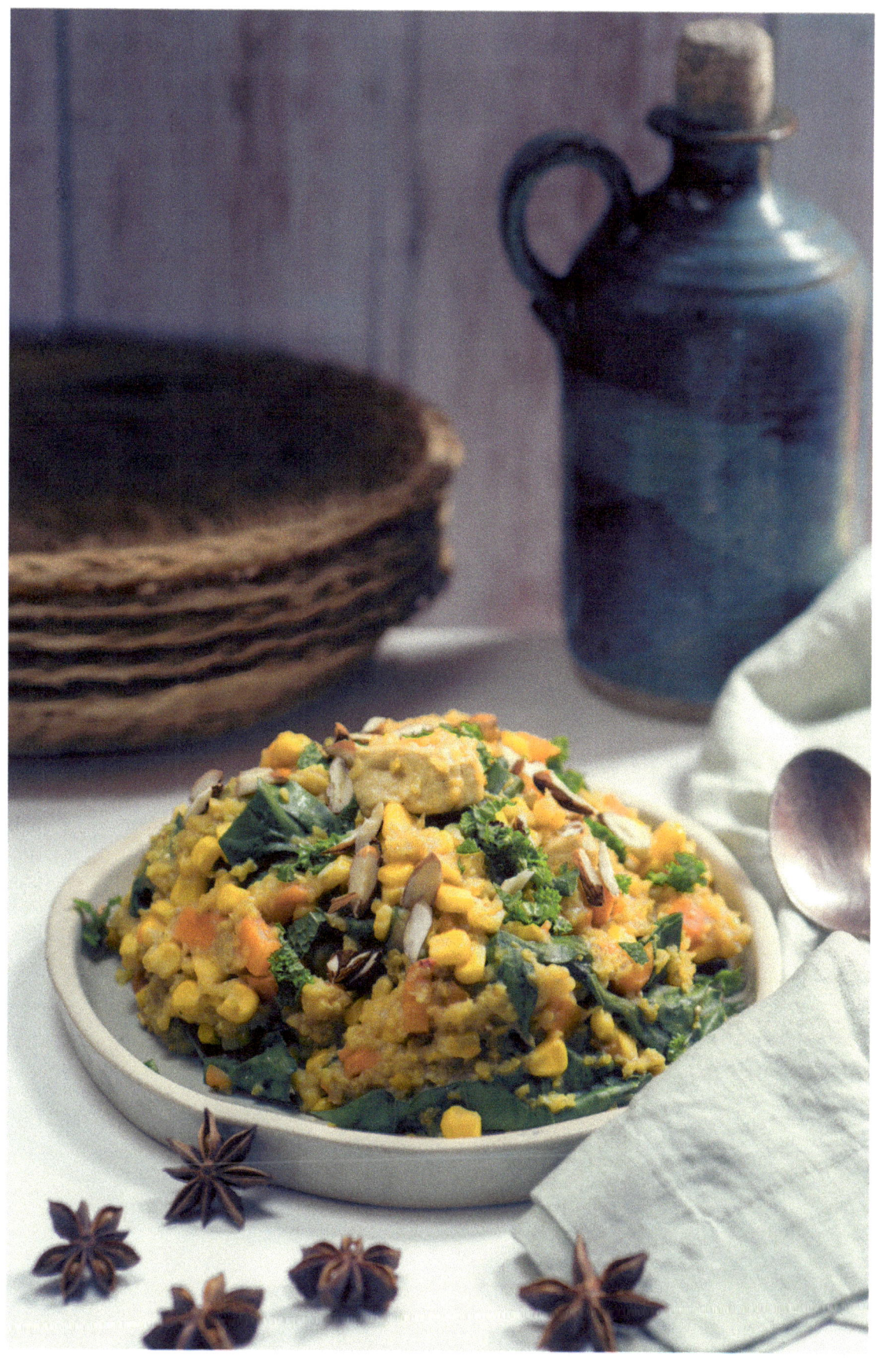

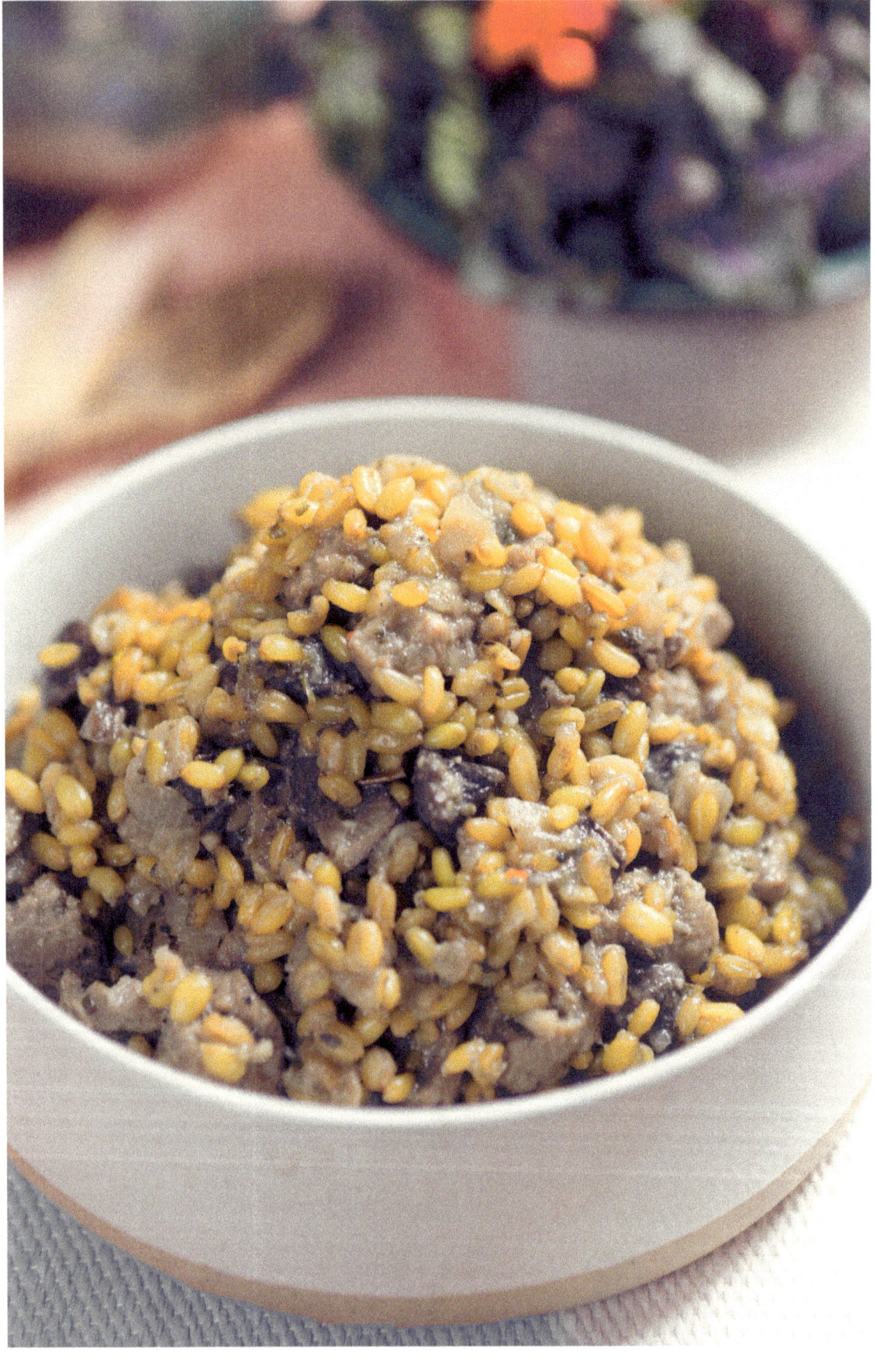

FREEKY RISOTTO

KCAL 266 | PROTEIN 19g | FAT 8.6g | CARBS 32g | SERVES 4

INGREDIENTS

1 cup freekeh

1 cup soy chunks

2 onions, chopped

2 cloves garlic, crushed

2 tbsp extra-virgin olive oil

pinch of salt

pinch of black pepper

2 tsp Italian herbs

1 tsp thyme

3 cups mushrooms, chopped

1 cup vegetable stock

1 cup light soy milk

METHOD

1. Pre-soak the freekeh and soy chunks overnight. Rinse thoroughly and drain until the water runs clear.

2. Sauté the onion and garlic in the olive oil. Add the salt, pepper and herbs. Add the freekeh little by little and sauté until the grains start to go translucent.

3. Add the mushrooms and soy chunks and sauté for 1 minute. Add the vegetable stock and soy milk.

4. Simmer for 30 minutes until the liquid is absorbed, leaving a smooth, creamy risotto. Freekeh remains chewy when cooked.

5. Serve with a side of salad.

Note

1. You can also substitute half of the cup of stock for an extra ½ cup of soy milk for a creamier texture.

LEMON-GLAZED TOFU STEAK

KCAL 396 | PROTEIN 25g | FAT 21g | CARBS 36g | SERVES 2

INGREDIENTS

400g firm tofu

For the glaze

1 lemon, juiced

1 stick lemongrass, finely chopped

1 tsp turmeric, grated

1-inch stick ginger, peeled and grated

1 tbsp extra-virgin olive oil

2 cloves garlic, crushed

pinch of salt and white pepper

For the salad

2 carrots, spiralled

1 radish, spiralled

1 zucchini, spiralled

5 spring onions, sliced

For the topping

2 tbsp seaweed

2 tbsp sweet soy sauce

10g sesame seeds, toasted

METHOD

1. **For the glaze** – Make a glaze from the lemon juice, lemongrass, grated turmeric, grated ginger, olive oil, crushed garlic, salt and pepper.

2. **For the tofu** – Rinse tofu and drain. Cut into two ½-inch slabs. Marinate in the glaze for at least 1 hour in the fridge. Rehydrate the seaweed in a small bowl.

3. **For the salad** – Prepare a salad of spiralled carrot, radish and zucchini using a spiralling machine and mix with the spring onions (setting some spring onions aside for the garnish).

4. Place tofu and glaze into an oven-proof dish and bake at medium temperature for 15 minutes or until it starts to turn brown.

5. Take the glazed tofu and place on the salad. Drizzle the glaze from the dish and the sweet soy sauce on top of the tofu steaks. Top with rehydrated seaweed, reserved spring onions and toasted sesame seeds to serve.

Note

1. If you don't have toasted sesame seeds you can make up a batch. Spread them on a non-stick baking tray and toast on low heat, tossing occasionally, for 8–10 minutes or until they turn golden. Make sure to monitor them as they can burn quickly. You can store them in a sealed jar for up to 3–6 months.

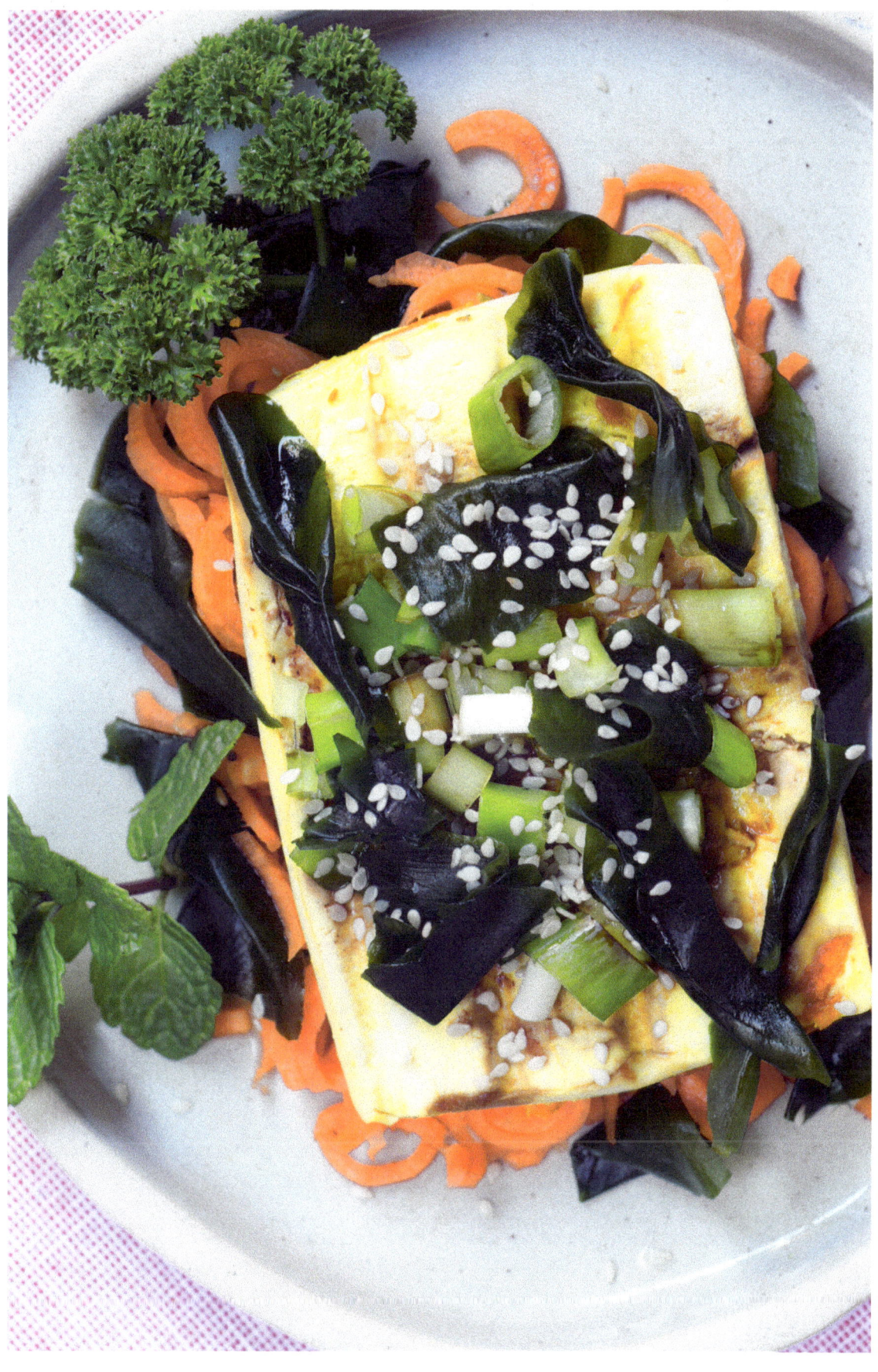

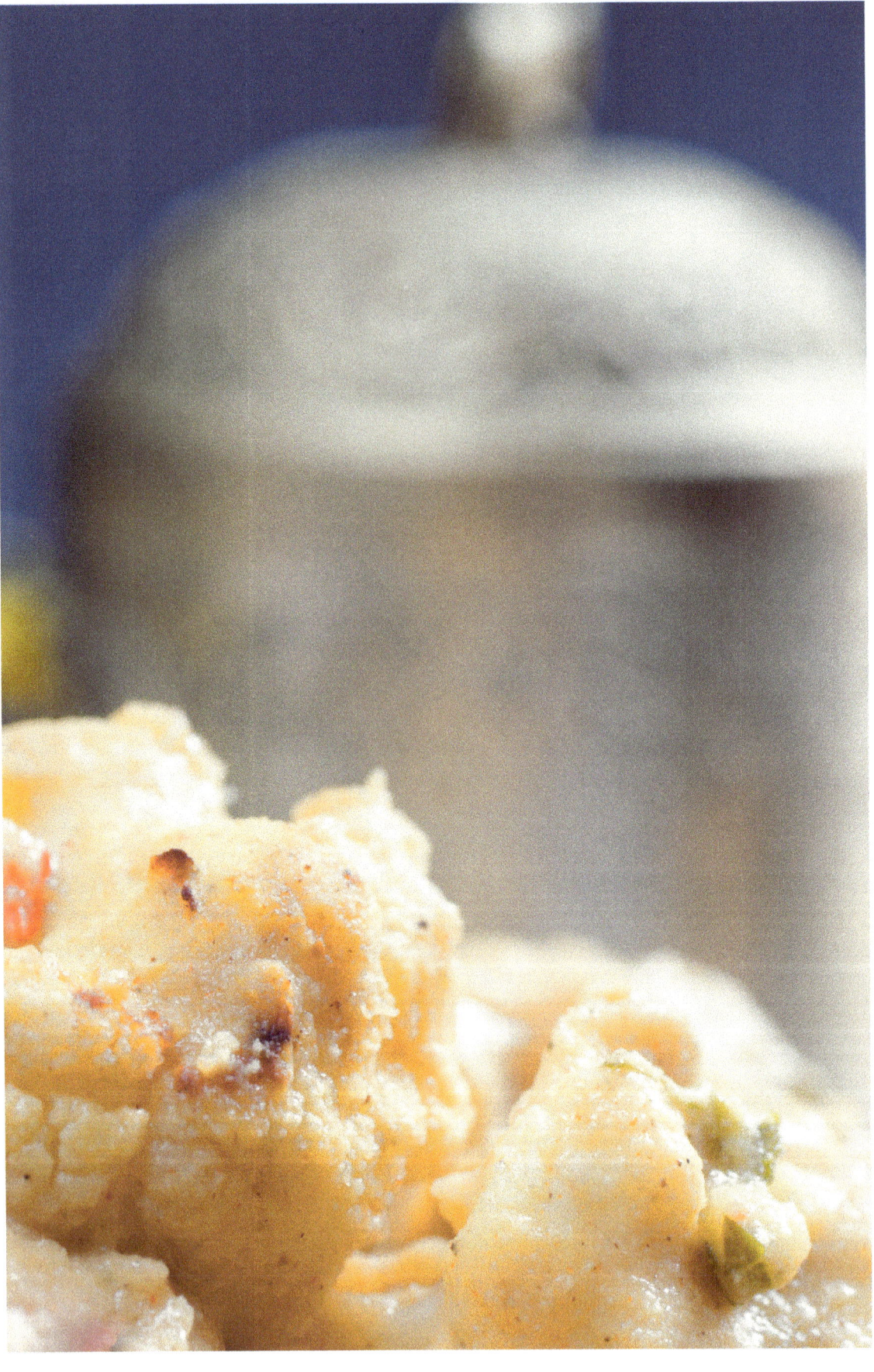

CAULIFLOWER QUESO

KCAL 108 | PROTEIN 7g | FAT 2.7g | CARBS 15g | SERVES 4

INGREDIENTS

1 cauliflower, separated into florets

For the queso sauce

2 cloves garlic

½ white onion

1 tomato

2 cups light soy milk

pinch of salt

pinch of black pepper

2 heaped tbsp nutritional yeast flakes

1 tbsp apple cider vinegar

1 tbsp cornflour

1 tbsp fresh coriander, chopped

1 tbsp fresh oregano, chopped

¼ tsp cumin powder

1 tsp smoked paprika

2 red chilli peppers, chopped

For the garnish

fresh parsley, chopped

METHOD

1. **For the cauliflower** – Place the cauliflower florets in boiling water with 1 tsp salt for 2–3 minutes off the heat.

2. **For the queso sauce** – Roughly chop the garlic, onion and tomato and blend together with the soy milk, salt and pepper, yeast flakes, vinegar and cornflour.

Stir the fresh herbs, spices and red chilli pepper into the sauce.

3. Transfer the cauliflower into a baking dish and pour the queso sauce over the cauliflower.

4. Bake in the oven on medium heat for 15–20 minutes or until the cauliflower starts to brown.

5. Serve with chopped fresh parsley to garnish.

SORGHUM BROCCOLI RISOTTO

KCAL 255 | PROTEIN 14g | FAT 5.9g | CARBS 42g | SERVES 4

INGREDIENTS

½ cup sorghum

1 onions, chopped

2 cloves garlic, crushed

1 tbsp extra-virgin olive oil

pinch of salt

pinch of white pepper

1¾ cups vegetable stock

3 cups broccoli, chopped

2 cups peas

1 tbsp vinegar

4 tbsp nutritional yeast flakes

1 tbsp rosemary

METHOD

1. Pre-soak the sorghum overnight. Rinse and drain.

2. Sauté the onion, garlic and sorghum in the oil with the salt and pepper for 2 minutes until translucent.

3. Add 1½ cups of the vegetable stock and simmer for 45–60 minutes or until the sorghum is soft but still chewy.

4. Add the broccoli and peas with the remaining stock, vinegar, yeast flakes and rosemary and simmer for 2–3 minutes until the broccoli is cooked.

5. Serve.

Notes

1. You can find and try different types of sorghum – in this recipe we have used red sorghum.

2. You could substitute broccoli with seasonal vegetables.

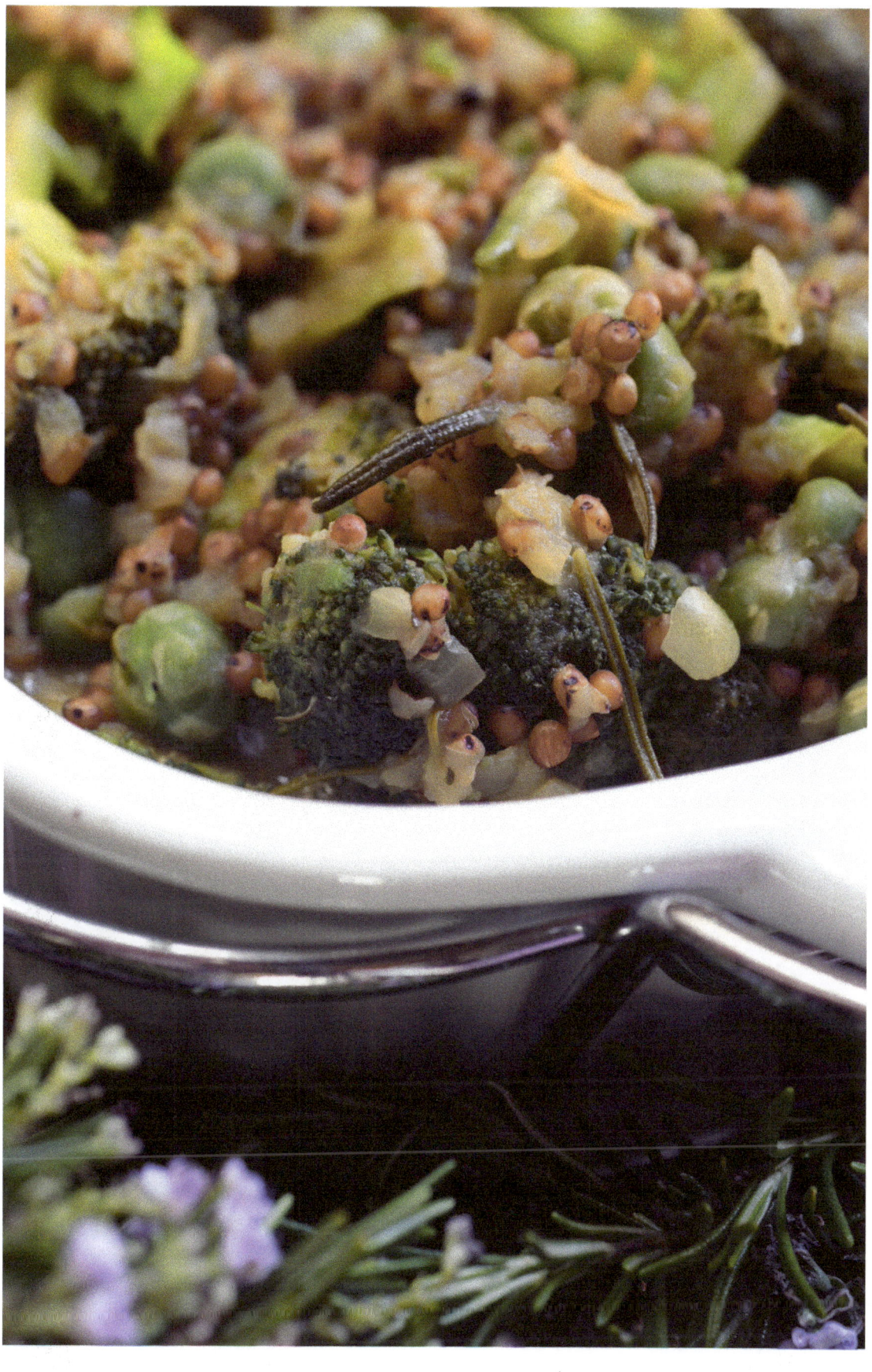

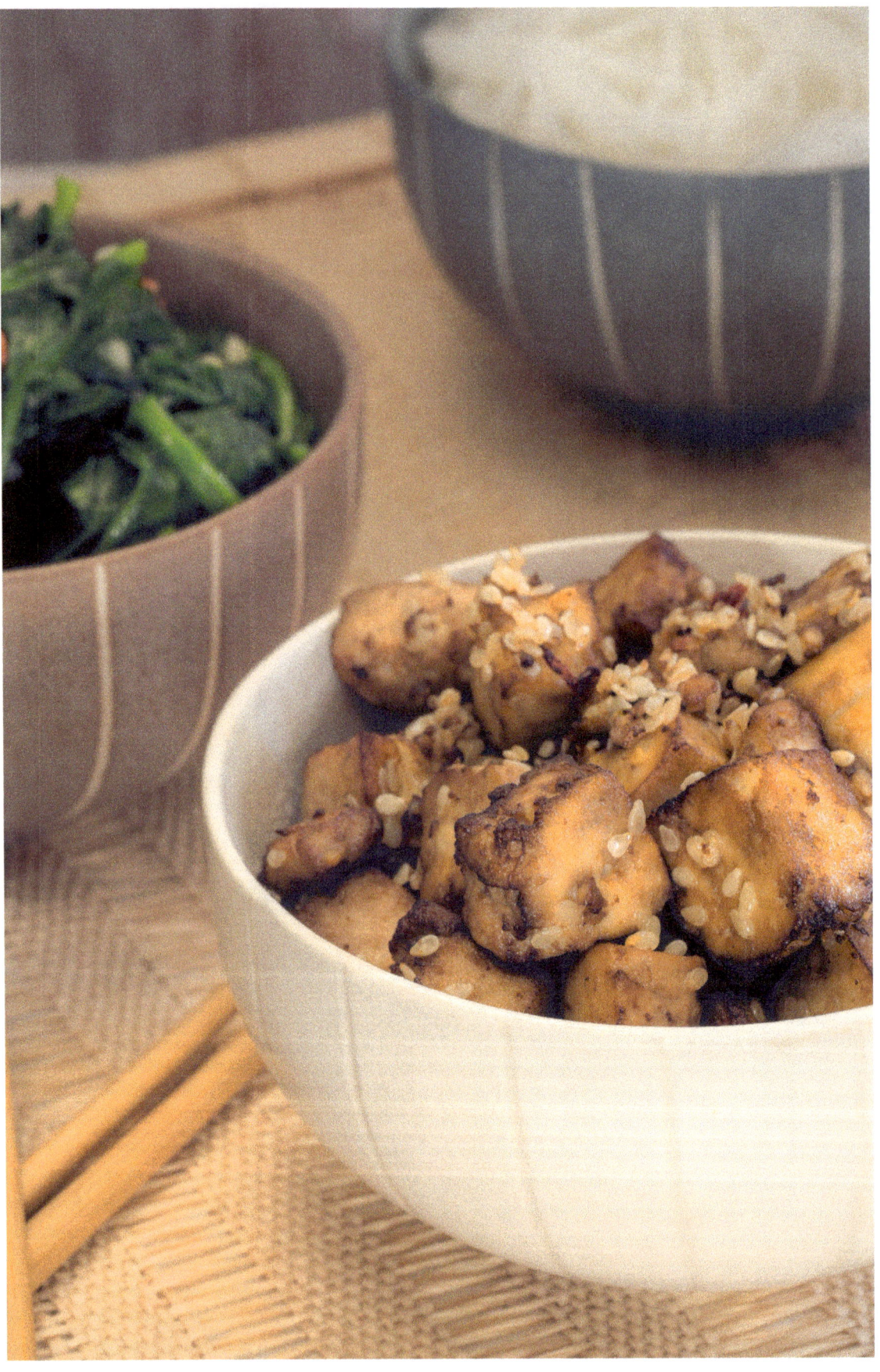

CHINESE TOFU

KCAL 268 | PROTEIN 22g | FAT 20g | CARBS 6.2g | SERVES 2

INGREDIENTS

400g extra-firm tofu

2 tbsp light soy sauce

1 tbsp extra-virgin olive oil

2 cloves garlic, crushed

1 tsp chilli powder

2 star anise pods

1-inch stick ginger, peeled and grated

For the garnish

1 tbsp toasted sesame seeds

METHOD

1. **For the tofu** – Rinse and drain the tofu and cut into cubes.

2. **For the marinade** – Mix the soy sauce, oil, garlic, chilli powder, star anise and grated ginger. Place the tofu in the marinade and leave for 2–3 hours in the fridge or overnight.

3. Take the tofu and marinade and place into a pan. Cook on medium heat for 8–10 minutes or until tofu is cooked and the sauce is thickened.

4. Remove star anise pods and serve with a garnish of toasted sesame seeds.

ROAST CARROT CUTLETS

KCAL 282 | PROTEIN 15g | FAT 14g | CARBS 28g | SERVES 4

INGREDIENTS

500g extra-firm tofu

8 carrots, sliced

2 red onions, sliced

1 sweet potato, thinly sliced

2 tbsp extra-virgin olive oil

For the marinade

'Lime and coriander marinade' (see recipe on page 111)

For the crumb

2 tbsp polenta

pinch of salt and black pepper or to taste

1 tsp smoked paprika

2 tbsp Italian herbs

½ tsp cayenne pepper

For the garnish

fresh parsley, chopped

METHOD

1. **For the tofu** – Make a marinade (we suggest the '*Lime and coriander marinade*' on page 111). Rinse and drain tofu and cut into slices. Marinate overnight.

2. **For the crumb** – Mix the polenta with salt, pepper, smoked paprika, Italian herbs and cayenne pepper.

3. Remove tofu, discard the marinade and coat directly with polenta crumb. Arrange on a baking tray.

4. Arrange the sliced vegetables on the tray alongside the cutlets.

5. Spray or brush the olive oil onto the vegetables.

6. Bake in the oven on medium heat for 25 minutes or until the carrots start to brown.

7. Serve with a sprinkle of fresh parsley.

Note

1. The nutritional information does not include the marinade.

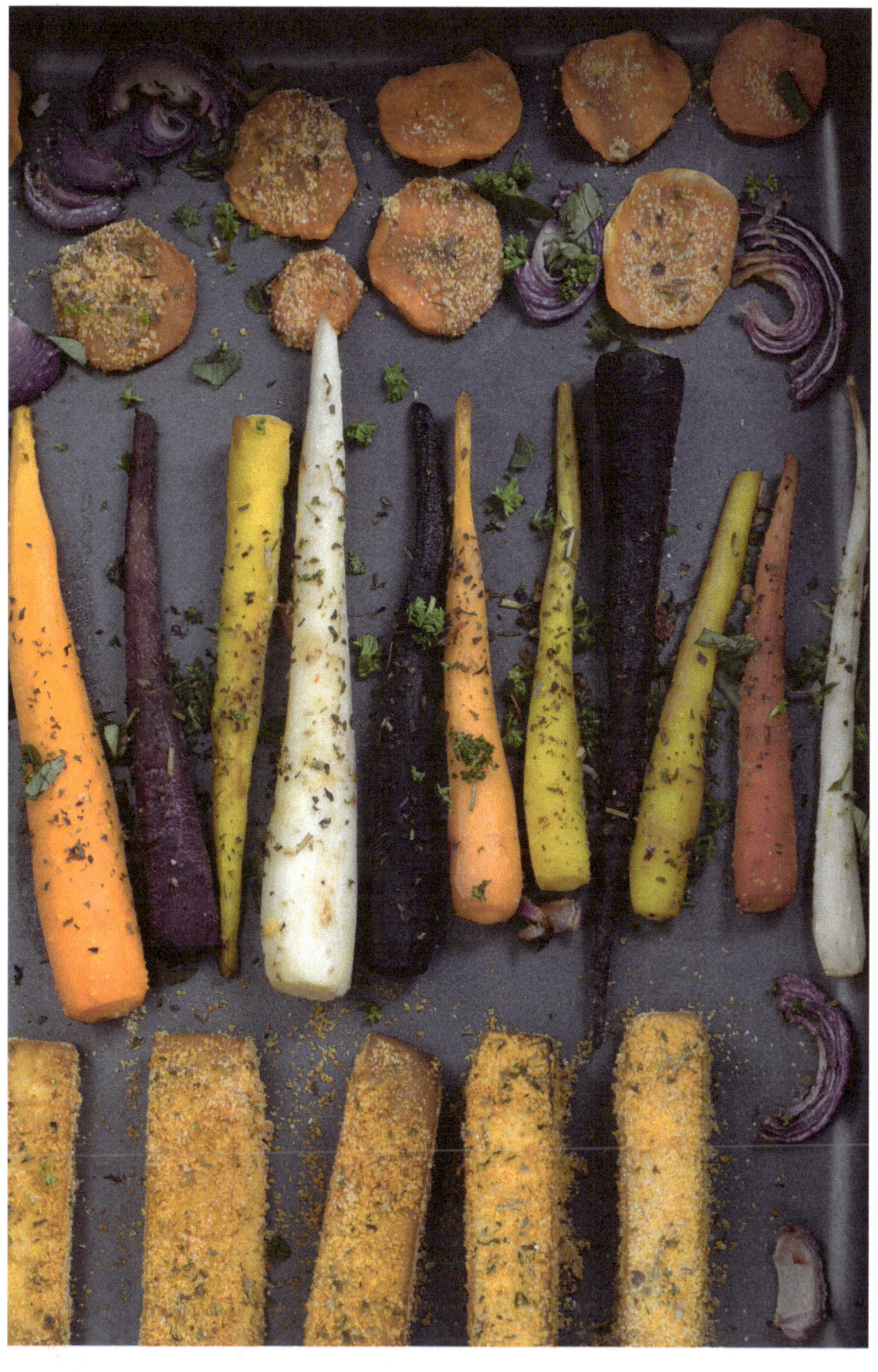

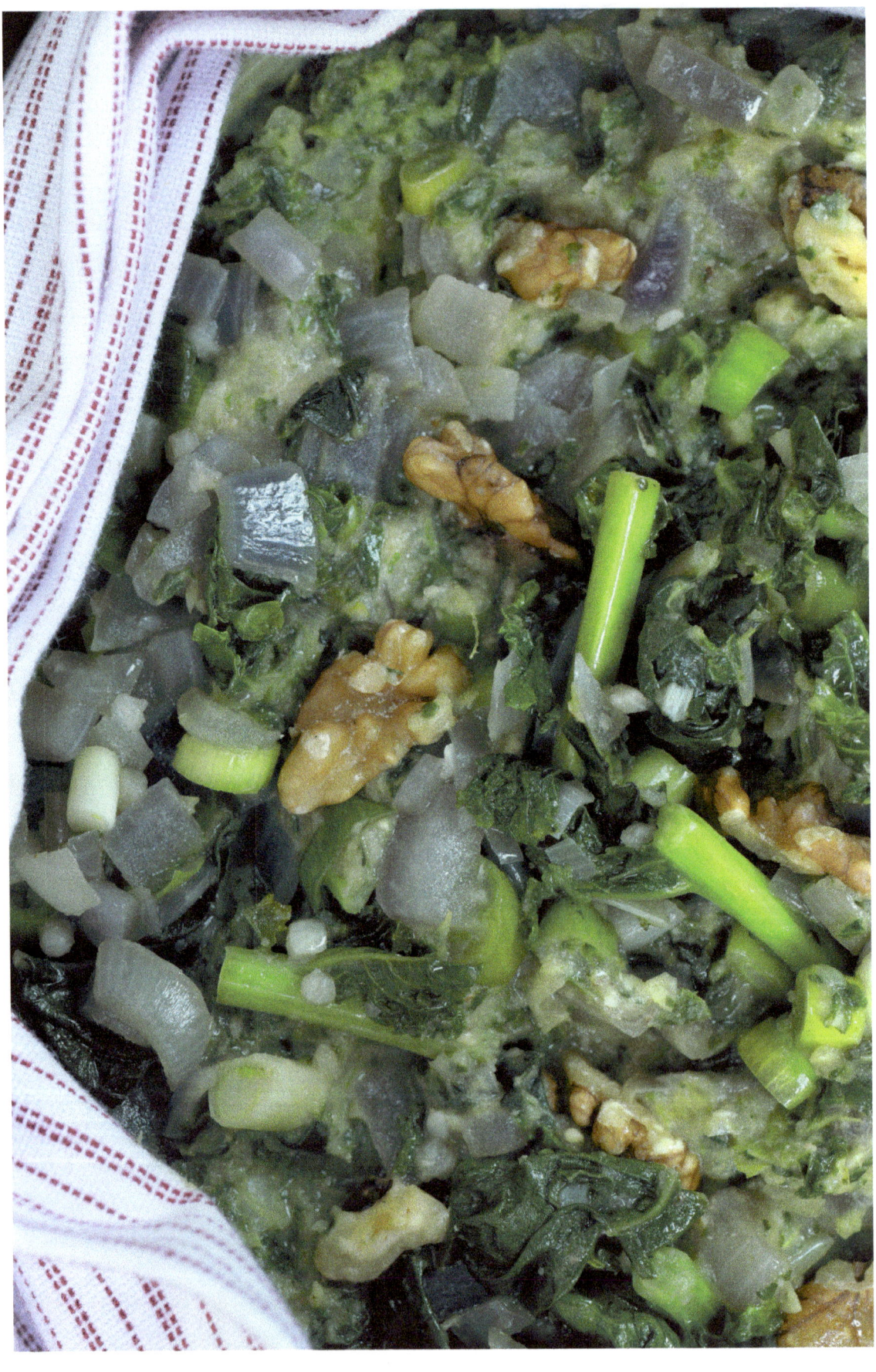

SWEET POTATO COLCANNON BOWL

KCAL 330 | PROTEIN 18g | FAT 11g | CARBS 47g | SERVES 4

INGREDIENTS

For the sweet potatoes

100g cannelloni beans

250g sweet potatoes, chopped

¼ cup light soy milk

6 tbsp nutritional yeast flakes

For the greens

1 onion, chopped

3 cloves garlic, crushed

1 leek, chopped

1 tbsp extra-virgin olive oil

pinch of salt or to taste

pinch of black pepper

4 cups kale or other greens, roughly chopped

To serve

5 green onions, sliced thinly

¼ cup walnuts, chopped

METHOD

1. Rinse and drain the beans.

2. **For the sweet potatoes** – Place the sweet potatoes in a pan of salted water and bring to the boil. Simmer for 10–15 minutes until the potatoes are soft.

Remove the sweet potatoes from the water, place in a bowl with the light soy milk and nutritional yeast flakes and mash together with the beans.

3. **For the greens** – Sauté the onion, garlic and leek in olive oil and seasoning until they start to turn brown. Add the kale and cook for 1–2 minutes.

4. Combine the sauté mixture into the sweet potatoes and stir to combine. Add the sliced green onions and walnuts and mix well. Season to taste and serve.

Note

1. Kale can be substituted with any greens and the vegetables can be substituted with seasonal vegetables that you have in your refrigerator – this recipe is great for using up leftover food in your kitchen.

CHEESY HERBED CAPSICUMS

KCAL 251 | PROTEIN 15g | FAT 8.5g | CARBS 34g | SERVES 4

INGREDIENTS

2 yellow capsicums (bell peppers)

1 tsp extra-virgin olive oil

20 almonds, sliced

For the filling

2 tsp cornflour

2 cups light soy milk

8 portobello mushrooms, chopped

1 tsp fresh thyme, chopped

1 tsp fresh parsley, chopped

1 tsp fresh oregano, chopped

150g sweetcorn kernels

4 tbsp nutritional yeast flakes

2 tbsp apple cider vinegar

2 tbsp fine couscous

pinch of salt

pinch of black pepper

METHOD

1. **For the capsicums** – Wash and halve lengthwise, scooping out the seeds. Place on a baking tray and lightly spray with the olive oil. Arrange the almonds on the baking tray. Set aside.

2. **For the filling** – Combine the cornflour with 2 tbsp of the soy milk and whisk with a fork until smooth. Add back to the rest of the soy milk and combine with the remaining ingredients. Season to taste.

3. Place the mixture in an oven-proof dish and place in the oven.

4. Bake the capsicums, almonds and mixture for 10–15 minutes on a low-medium heat until they start to turn golden. Watch the almonds as they can burn quickly.

5. Remove from the oven and arrange capsicums on a serving plate. Spoon the filling into the capsicums and top with the almonds.

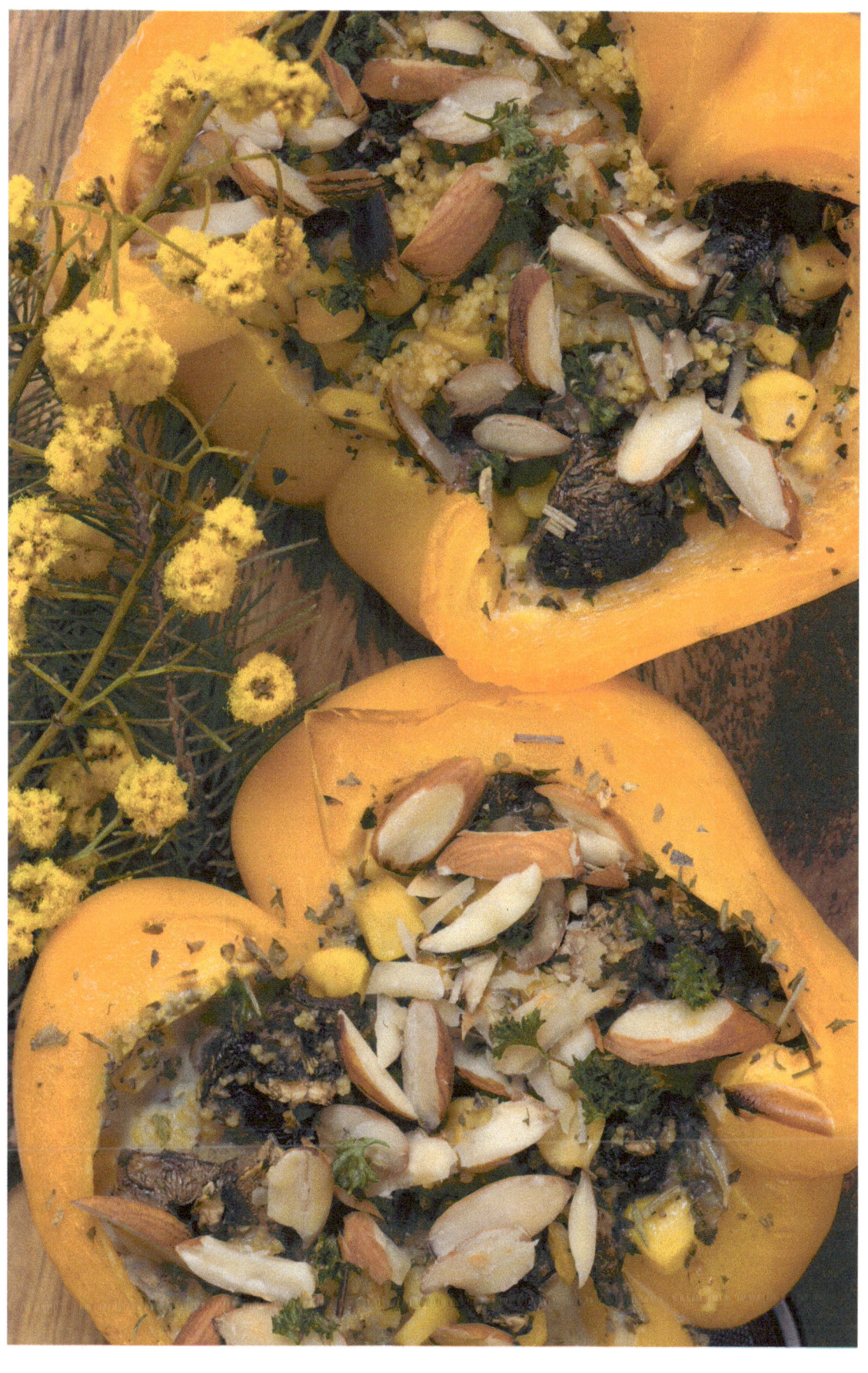

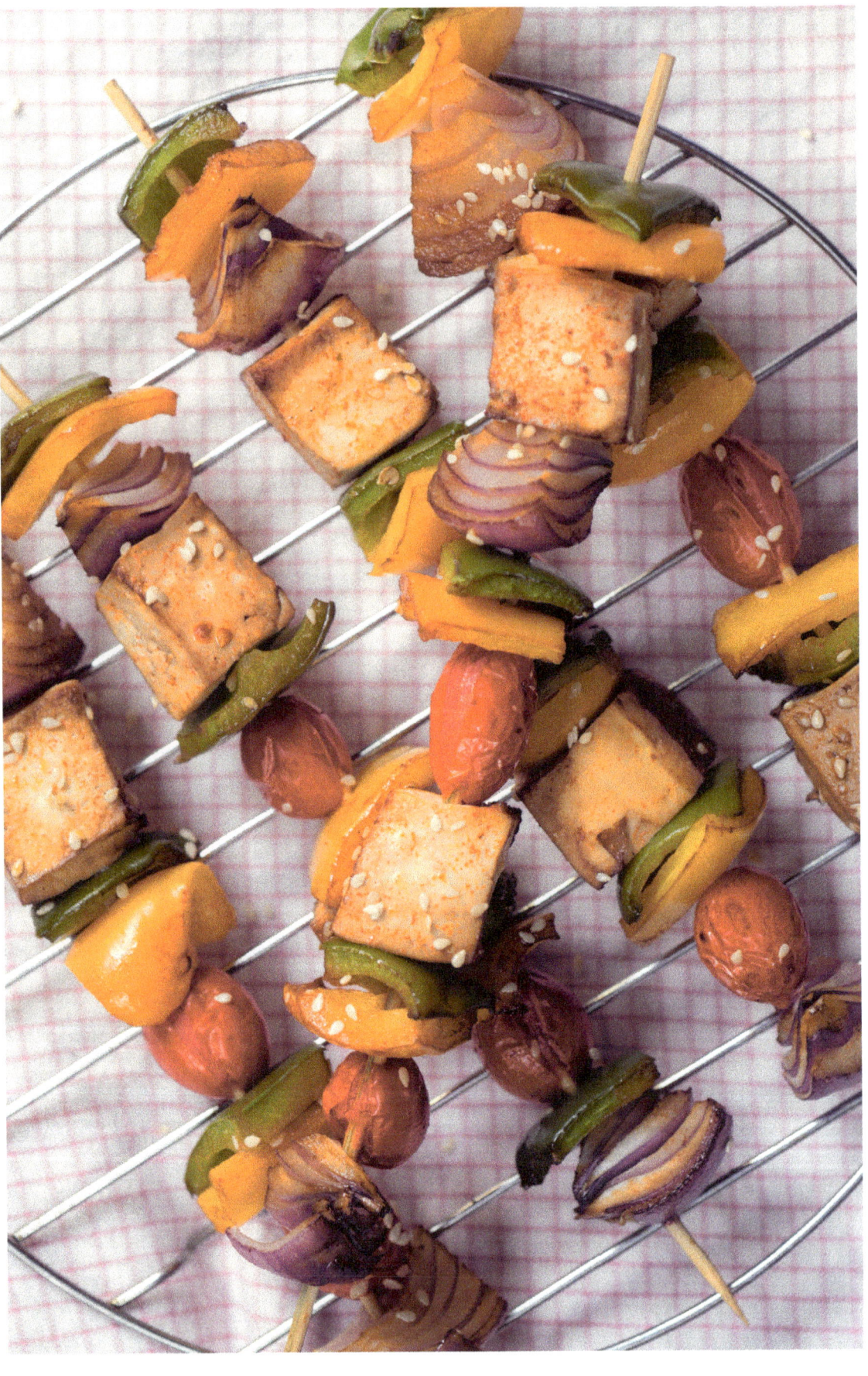

TOFU SKEWERS

KCAL 151 | PROTEIN 12g | FAT 9g | CARBS 9g | SERVES 5 (2 skewers per serve)

INGREDIENTS

500g extra-firm tofu

1 tbsp extra-virgin olive oil

1 tbsp light soy sauce

1 tbsp sweet soy sauce

1 tbsp vinegar

1 tsp ginger powder

1 tsp smoked paprika

½ tsp chilli powder (optional)

½ tsp cayenne pepper

20 baby tomatoes

1 yellow capsicum (bell pepper), cubed

1 small red onion, cubed

1 tbsp sesame seeds, toasted

METHOD

1. Rinse and drain the tofu. Cut into cubes.

2. Mix the oil, light soy sauce, sweet soy sauce, vinegar and spices in a bowl and marinate the tofu cubes in the mixture in the fridge for 2–3 hours or overnight.

3. Thread the chopped vegetables and tofu sequentially onto skewers.

4. Pour the remaining marinade over the skewers and grill or barbecue for 5–6 minutes or until golden brown, turning regularly.

5. Serve sprinkled with toasted sesame seeds.

Note

1. Toasted sesame seeds can be stored in a jar for 3–6 months so it is a good idea to make a batch to keep in your pantry. Just lay the sesame seeds on a baking tray and toast on low heat for 5–10 minutes until they start to turn golden brown.

TERIYAKI TOFU

KCAL 236 | PROTEIN 16g | FAT 11g | CARBS 20g | SERVES 4

INGREDIENTS

500g firm tofu

4 tbsp mirin

1–2 fresh red chilli peppers, sliced

1 tsp cornflour

1-inch stick fresh ginger, peeled and grated

2 tbsp green onions, sliced

pinch of salt or to taste

pinch of white pepper or to taste

For the marinade

2 tbsp light soy sauce

2 tbsp sweet soy sauce

2 tbsp rice wine vinegar

2 cloves garlic, crushed

1 tsp sesame oil

For the garnish

1 tbsp toasted sesame seeds

METHOD

1. Combine the light soy sauce, sweet soy sauce, rice wine vinegar, crushed garlic and sesame oil.

2. Rinse, drain and cut the tofu into cubes. Marinate for 2–3 hours or overnight.

3. Place the tofu and marinade into an oven-proof dish. Add the mirin, sliced red chilli pepper, cornflour, fresh ginger and green onions. Add salt and pepper to taste.

4. Bake on medium heat for 10-15 minutes and serve garnished with toasted sesame seeds.

Notes

1. Fresh red chilli peppers can be substituted with chilli powder.

2. Sesame oil can be substituted with extra-virgin olive oil.

3. Fresh ginger can be substituted with 1 tsp ginger powder.

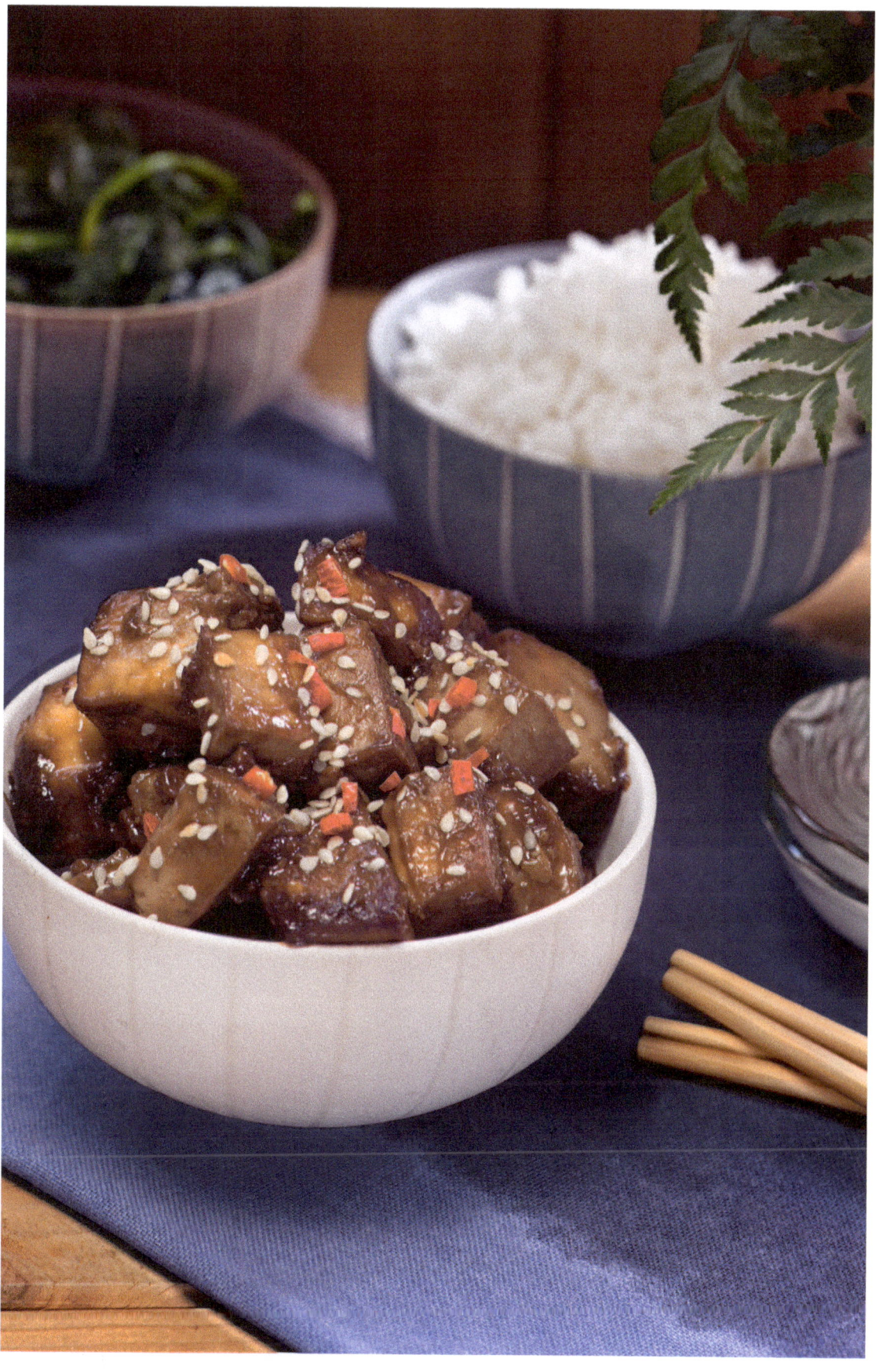

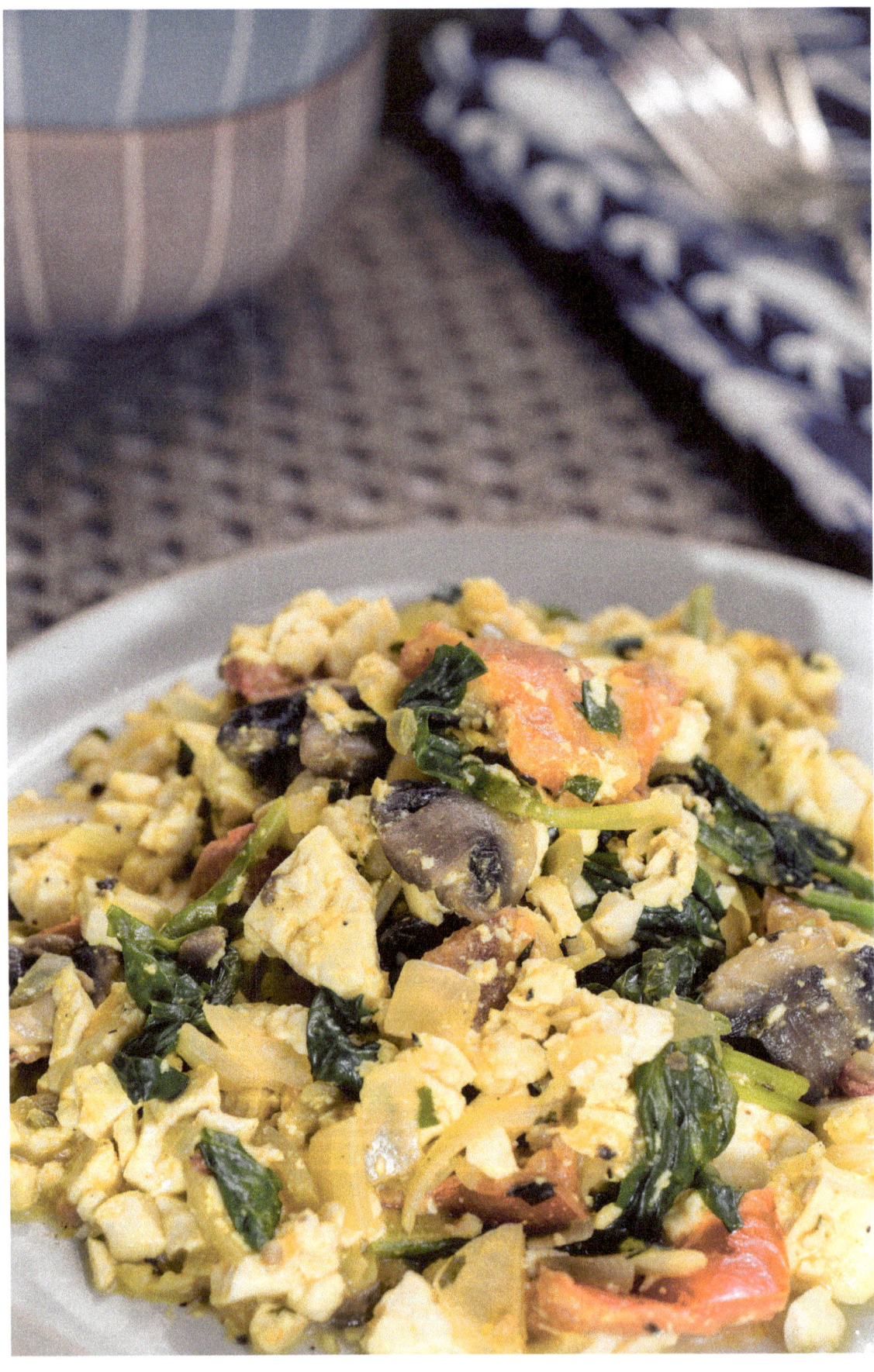

TOFU MEDITERRANEAN SCRAMBLE

KCAL 287 | PROTEIN 24g | FAT 16g | CARBS 20g | SERVES 2

INGREDIENTS

300g semi-firm tofu

¼ tsp salt

2 tbsp nutritional yeast flakes

2 shallots, chopped

1 clove garlic

1 tbsp extra-virgin olive oil

2 pinches black salt or to taste

pinch of black pepper

4 medium fresh mushrooms

¼ tsp turmeric

½ tsp dried oregano or Italian herbs

1 tomato, chopped

1 tbsp apple cider vinegar

2 cups fresh spinach, chopped

For the garnish

1 tbsp fresh basil, chopped

METHOD

1. Rinse tofu and drain. Crumble the tofu and mix with the salt and nutritional yeast flakes and set aside.

2. Sauté the shallots and garlic in the olive oil with black salt and pepper. Add the mushrooms, turmeric and herbs and cook until golden brown.

3. Add the tomato, apple cider vinegar and tofu to the pan, bring to simmer and cover, switching off heat. Let it stand for 2–3 minutes.

4. Open the lid and stir in spinach. Close lid and let it stand for another 2–3 minutes to wilt the spinach.

5. Serve the scramble with a garnish of fresh basil.

Notes

1. Feel free to add more seasonal veggies to this dish – another dish great for using up leftovers in your refrigerator.

2. If you don't have black salt, substitute with regular salt.

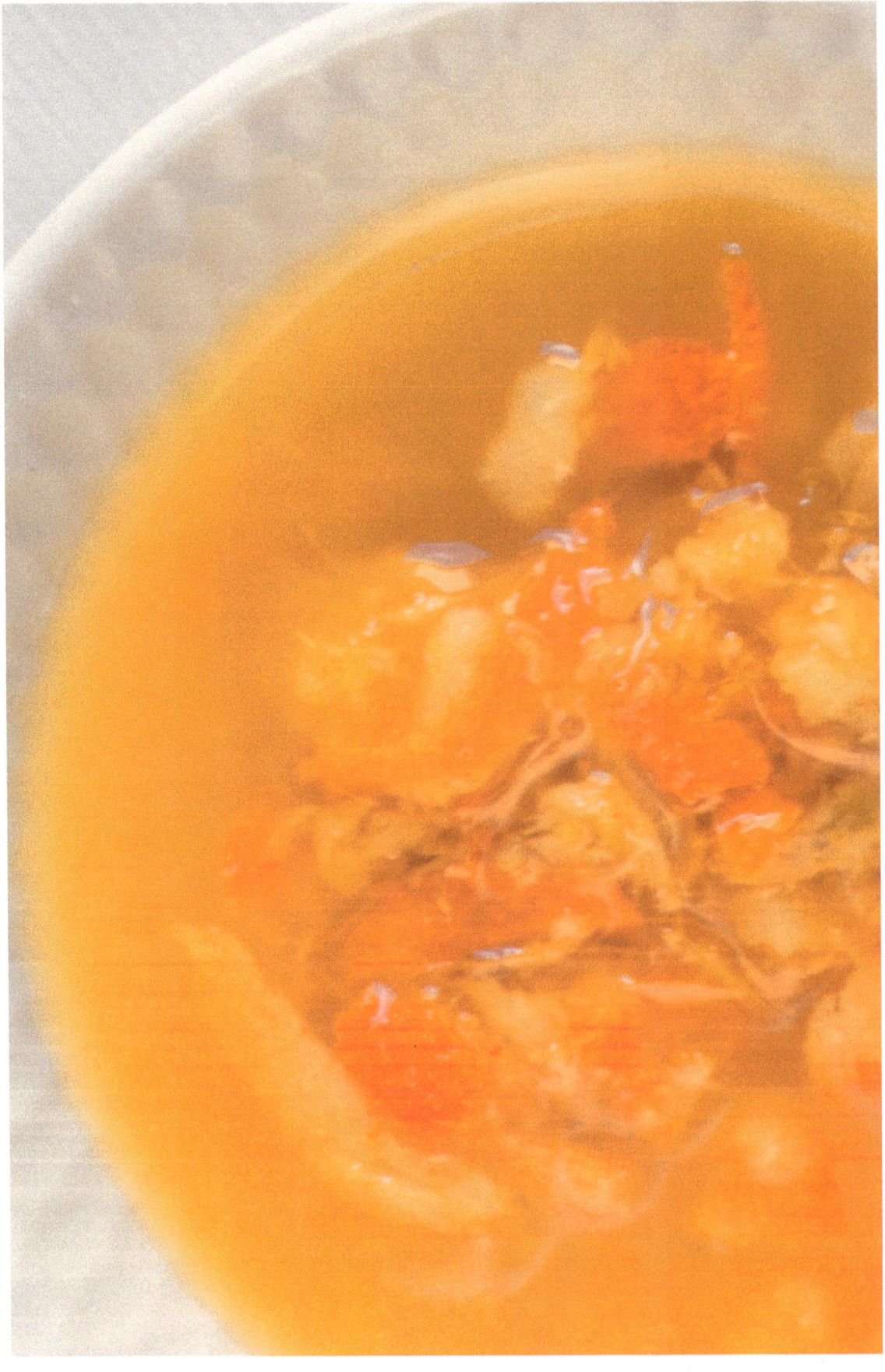

MARINADES

The secret to enjoying tofu is the marinade – and we have created five marinade recipes here to inspire you. They are not intended to be full dishes on their own but rather liquid mixtures in which you can steep your tofu before cooking to infuse it with flavours. The quantity shown in each recipe is enough for 250–300g tofu.

To prepare the tofu for the marinade, you can choose to 'press' the tofu to extract as much water as possible. You can do this by rinsing and draining the tofu, placing it on a rack that sits on a tray and then placing a chopping board on top of the tofu. Weigh down the chopping board and let it stand for 10–15 minutes so that excess water drains out.

An alternative method is to freeze the tofu (firm tofu works best) in a freezer bag for an hour or so until frozen. Defrost and drain the tofu before marinating. The process of freezing creates pockets in the tofu that readily absorb flavours and also gives the tofu more texture.

To use the marinades, prepare and combine the ingredients as instructed and place the liquid into a food storage box. Cut the tofu into the required size, for example slices or cubes. Then carefully place the tofu into the storage box with the marinade, seal and place in the refrigerator for 6–8 hours or overnight.

When you are ready to cook the tofu, use or discard the marinade as directed by the recipe.

TOMATO & CHILLI MARINADE

KCAL 66 | PROTEIN 2.3g | FAT 0.5g | CARBS 15g | SERVES n/a

INGREDIENTS

- 2 tomatoes, roughly chopped
- 1 white onion, peeled and roughly chopped
- 2 cloves garlic, peeled
- 2 fresh chilli peppers, roughly chopped
- pinch of salt
- pinch of black pepper
- 1 tbsp lemon juice
- 1 tbsp apple cider vinegar

METHOD

1. Combine all the ingredients in a blender.

2. Blend until smooth.

3. Use to marinate by placing the tofu in a food container with the marinade in the refrigerator.

Note

1. The fresh chilli peppers can be substituted with 1 tsp cayenne pepper.

GARLIC & GINGER MARINADE

KCAL 29 | PROTEIN 0.9g | FAT 0.2g | CARBS 5.2g | SERVES n/a

INGREDIENTS

2 tbsp apple cider vinegar

2 tbsp water

2-inch stick ginger, peeled

3 cloves garlic

pinch of black salt

pinch of black pepper

¼ tsp mustard

METHOD

1. Combine all the ingredients in a small blender.

2. Blend until smooth.

3. Use to marinate by placing the tofu in a food container with the marinade in the refrigerator.

Note

1. If you don't have black salt go ahead and use regular salt.

SPICED WARM MARINADE

KCAL 170 | PROTEIN 4.5g | FAT 3.3g | CARBS 36g | SERVES n/a

INGREDIENTS

2 tbsp sweet soy sauce

2 tbsp light soy sauce

1 tbsp apple cider vinegar

2 cloves garlic, peeled

3 star anise pods

5 clove pods

3 cardamom pods

1 tsp cayenne pepper

½ tsp turmeric

1-inch stick fresh ginger, peeled

½ tsp nutmeg

pinch of black pepper

METHOD

1. **Using a blender** – Combine all the ingredients in a small blender and blend until smooth.

Using a spice bag – Some recipes may call for the star anise, clove and cardamom pods to be placed in a spice bag for cooking.

2. Use to marinate by placing the tofu in a food container with the marinade in the refrigerator.

SWEET & SOUR MARINADE

KCAL 118 | PROTEIN 2.4g | FAT 0.2g | CARBS 29g | SERVES n/a

INGREDIENTS

- 2 tbsp sweet soy sauce
- 2 tbsp light soy sauce
- 1 fresh chilli pepper, roughly chopped
- 1 tbsp tamarind extract
- 2 tbsp apple cider vinegar

METHOD

1. Combine all the ingredients in a small blender.

2. Blend until smooth.

3. Use to marinate by placing the tofu in a food container with the marinade in the refrigerator.

Note

1. If you don't have tamarind extract, substitute with 2 tbsp lemon juice.

LEMON MARINADE

KCAL 106 | PROTEIN 2.4g | FAT 1.1g | CARBS 27g | SERVES n/a

INGREDIENTS

2 tbsp lemon juice

2 tbsp water

1 stick lemongrass, roughly chopped

2 cloves garlic, peeled

1-inch stick ginger, peeled

1-inch stick turmeric, peeled

1-inch stick galangal, peeled (optional)

pinch of salt

pinch of black pepper

METHOD

1. Combine all the ingredients in a small blender.

2. Blend until smooth.

3. Use to marinate by placing the tofu in a food container with the marinade in the refrigerator.

Note

1. ¼ tsp turmeric powder can be substituted for the fresh turmeric.

LIME & CORIANDER MARINADE

KCAL 58 | PROTEIN 4g | FAT 1.2g | CARBS 10g | SERVES n/a

INGREDIENTS

1 lime, juiced

pinch of black salt

2 pinches black pepper

1 clove garlic, peeled

1-inch stick ginger, peeled

½ tsp nutmeg

1 tsp cumin seeds

1-inch stick turmeric, peeled

¼ cup fresh coriander, roughly chopped

METHOD

1. Combine all the ingredients in a blender.

2. Blend until smooth.

3. Use to marinate by placing the tofu in a food container with the marinade in the refrigerator.

Notes

1. ¼ tsp turmeric powder can be substituted for the fresh turmeric.

2. If you don't have black salt go ahead and use regular salt.

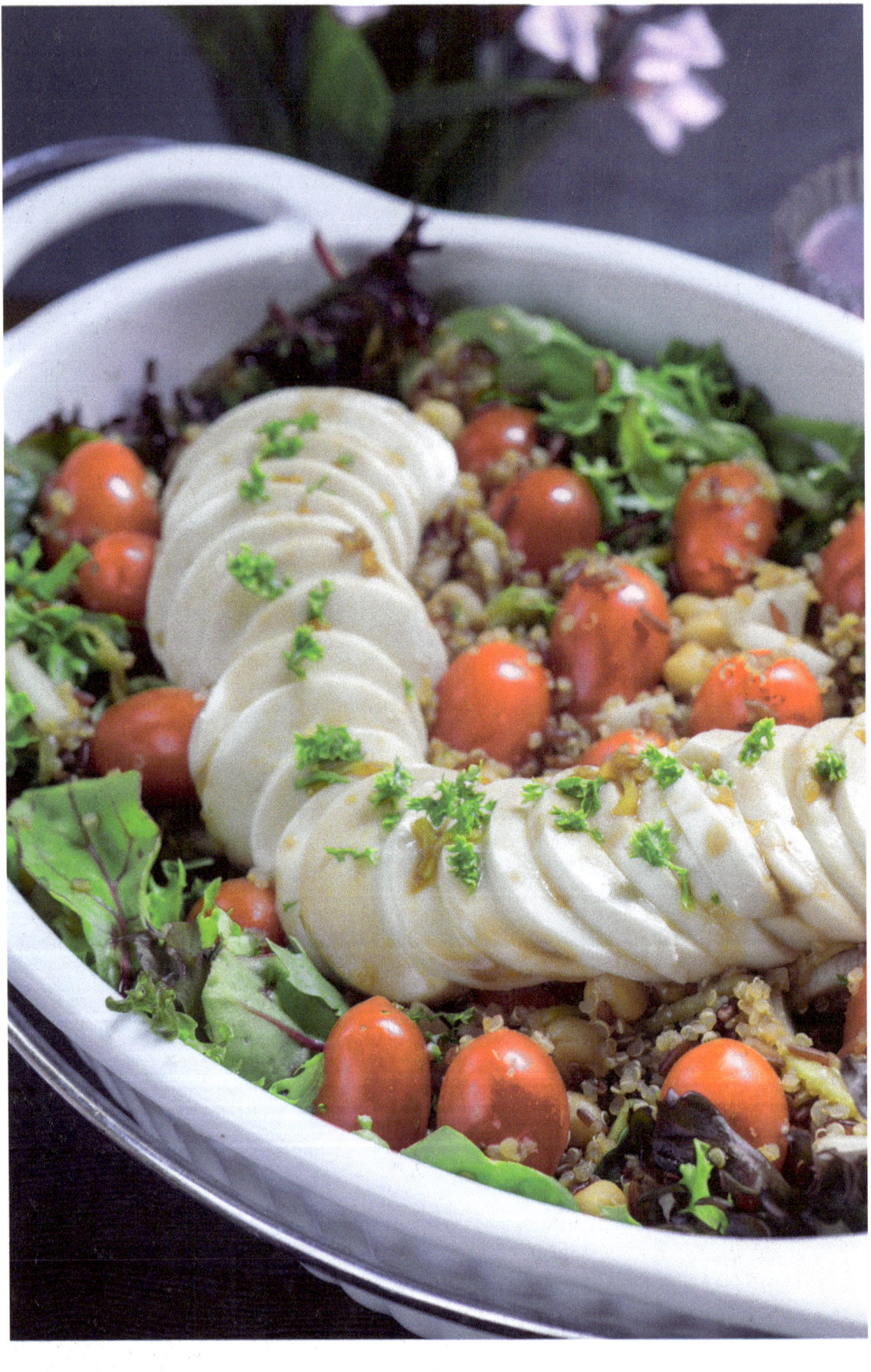

SALADS

With a combination of whole grains, legumes, seeds and proteins, a salad can be the perfect main course. Healthy, nutritious and full of protein, there are infinite combinations of flavours and textures that you can create. Start with these recipes as a source of inspiration.

Salads are also great for lunch boxes as you can pop them into the fridge and don't need to re-heat them before eating. If you are taking your salad with you in a lunch box it's a good idea to pack the salad dressing separately and toss directly before eating for maximum freshness.

These salad recipes together with their dressings provide at least 20% of their calories from protein – if you are substituting ingredients be sure to check the nutritional content as oil-based dressings can easily rack up the calories.

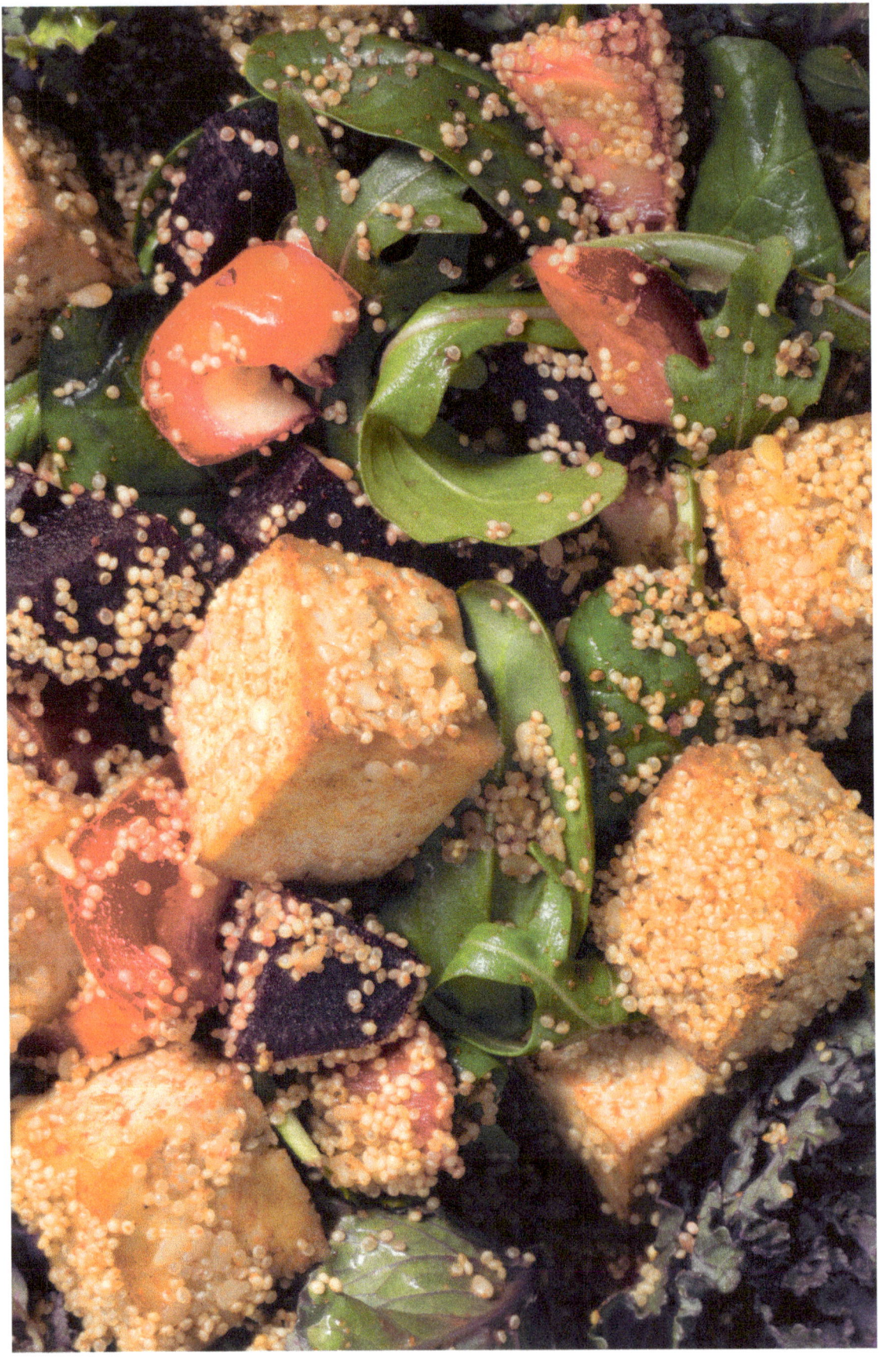

AMARANTH TOFU SALAD WITH LEMON DRESSING

KCAL 232 | PROTEIN 16g | FAT 11g | CARBS 23g | SERVES 4

INGREDIENTS

400g extra-firm tofu, cubed

For the marinade

2 tbsp light soy sauce

2 tbsp sweet soy sauce

2 cloves garlic, crushed

For the crumb

1 tbsp coconut flour

4 tbsp amaranth

4 tbsp sesame seeds, toasted

1 tsp Italian herbs

2 tsp smoked sweet paprika

½ tsp salt

For the salad

4 cups mixed salad

For the lemon dressing

½ cup lemon juice

pinch of salt

2 tbsp Dijon mustard

METHOD

1. **For the tofu** – Mix together the ingredients for the marinade. Rinse and drain the tofu, place in the refrigerator with the marinade for at least 2–3 hours.

2. **For the crumb** – Mix a crumb mixture using the coconut flour, amaranth, sesame seeds, herbs, spices and salt in a bowl.

3. Drain the tofu and discard the marinade. Press the tofu cubes directly into the crumb mixture to coat.

4. Bake the tofu on medium heat, turning once, for 15 minutes or until golden. Let cool and set aside.

5. **For the salad** – Wash, drain and prepare the salad vegetables. Prepare a salad dressing by mixing together the lemon juice, salt and mustard.

6. Toss the salad in the dressing and add the tofu cubes to serve.

PEARL COUSCOUS SPINACH SALAD

KCAL 239 | PROTEIN 14g | FAT 14g | CARBS 23g | SERVES 6

INGREDIENTS

For the tofu and couscous

400g firm tofu

2 cloves garlic, crushed

2 shallots, chopped

½ tsp nutmeg

½ tsp ginger powder

4 tbsp yeast flakes

pinch of salt and black pepper

3 tbsp extra-virgin olive oil

1 cup pearl couscous

1 cup vegetable stock

2 tbsp apple cider vinegar

For the salad

5 cups spinach

4 tomatoes, sliced

1 cucumber, spiralled

¼ cup olives

1 red onion, sliced

10 fresh mint leaves, chopped

2 tbsp fresh parsley, chopped

For the dressing
'French vinaigrette' (see page 126)

For the marinade
'Spiced warm marinade' (see page 108)

METHOD

1. **For the tofu** – Rinse the tofu and cut into ½-inch cubes. Marinate for 2–3 hours or overnight in the refrigerator. We recommend *'Spiced warm marinade'* from page 108.

2. Remove the tofu and discard the marinade.

3. **For the couscous** – Sauté the garlic, shallots, spices, yeast flakes, seasoning and tofu with the oil and then add the couscous incrementally and cook for 2–3 minutes.

4. When the couscous has browned add the vegetable stock and apple cider vinegar and cook until liquid has evaporated. Check the couscous is cooked – it should be firm but soft. If necessary add more water and simmer until cooked.

5. **For the salad** – Toss the prepared vegetables and herbs in the dressing (we recommend *'French vinaigrette'* on page 126). Add the couscous tofu mixture on top and serve.

Notes

1. The nutritional information does not include the salad dressing.

2. You can substitute the spinach with mixed greens of your choice.

3. 'Pearl couscous' is also called 'Israeli couscous'.

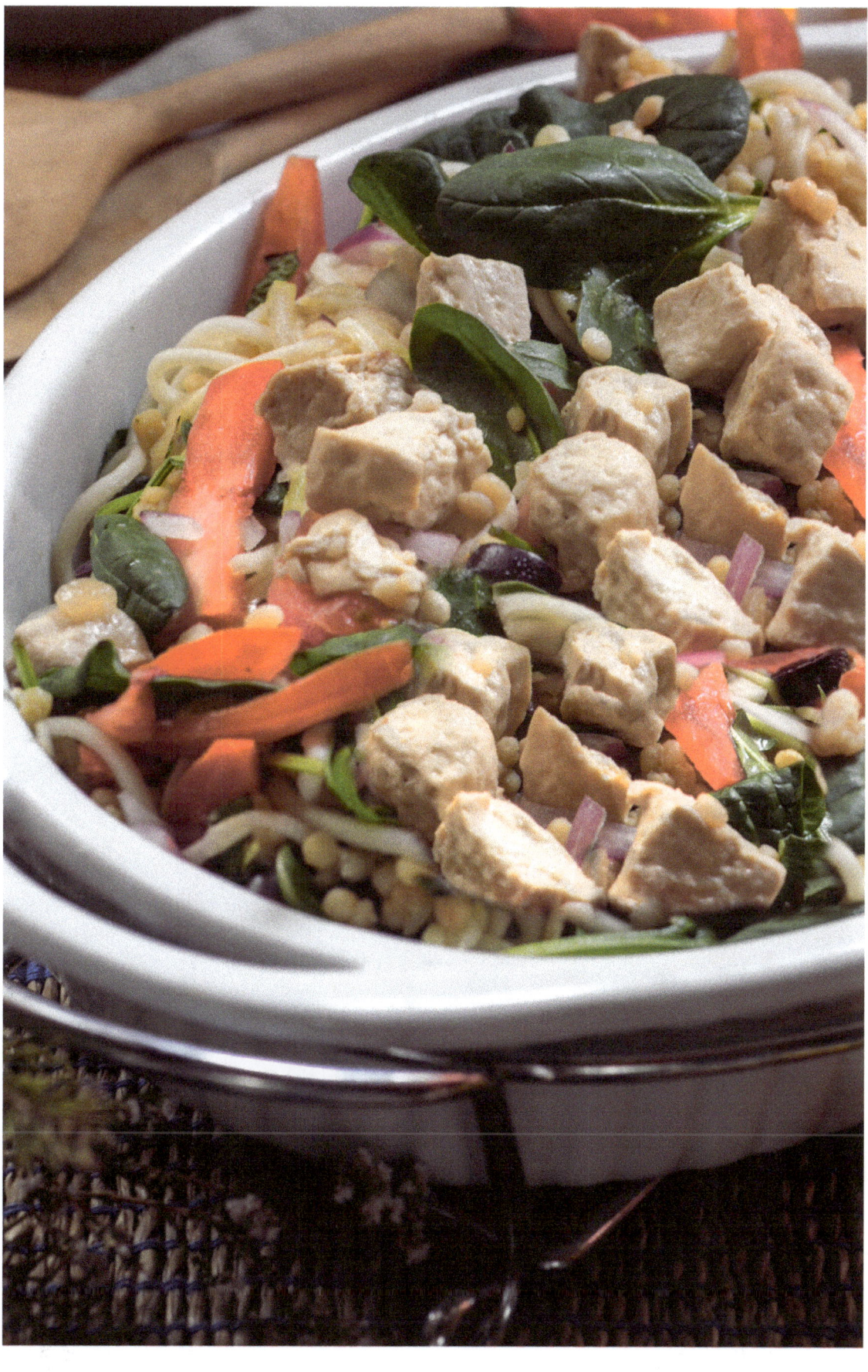

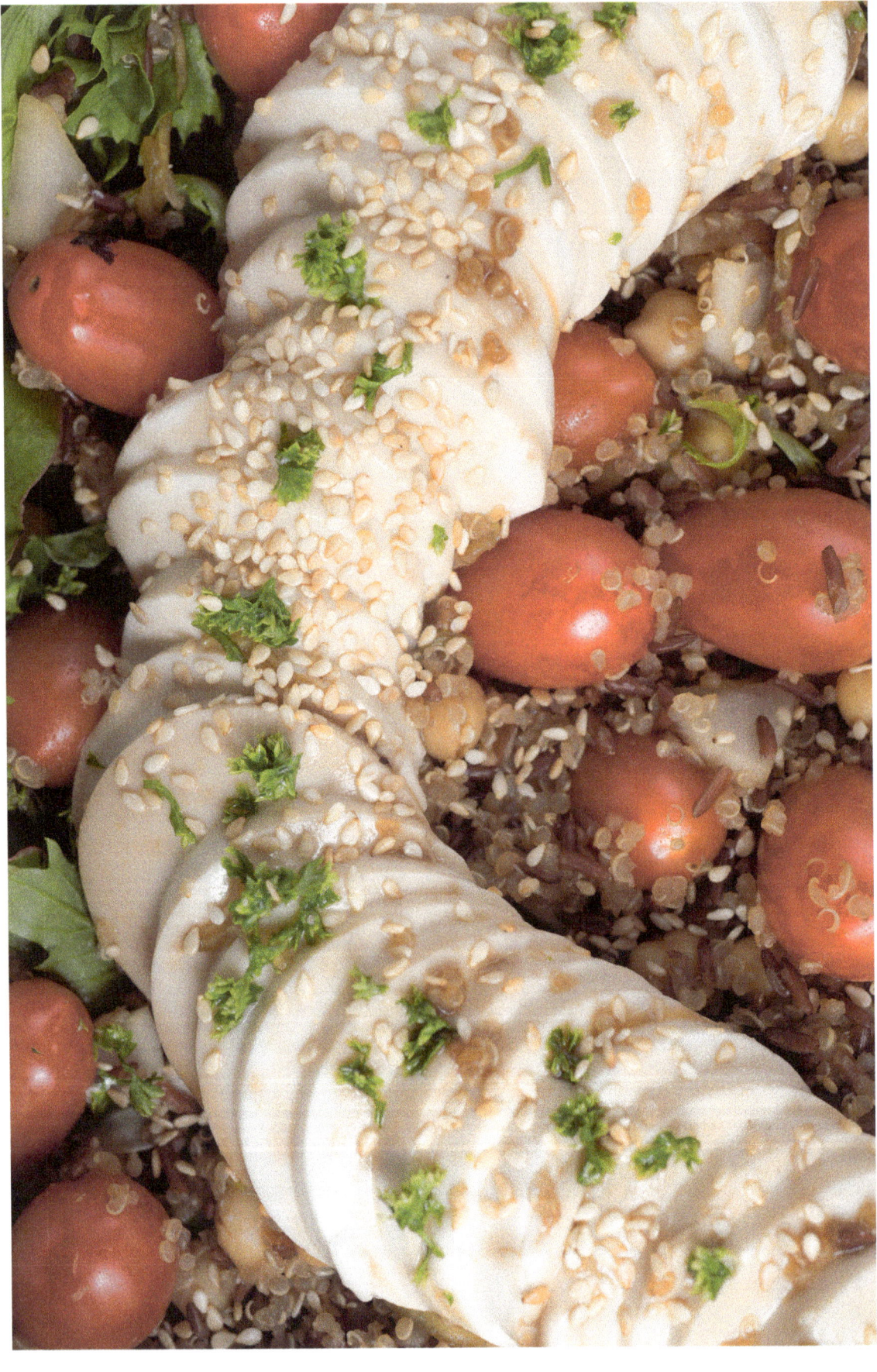

QUINOA & RED RICE MISO SALAD

KCAL 270 | PROTEIN 14g | FAT 8.8g | CARBS 39g | SERVES 4

INGREDIENTS

5 cups mixed greens

1 cup cherry tomatoes

¼ daikon radish

300g silken tofu

For the grains

115g cooked chickpeas (or 50g dried chickpeas)

¼ cup quinoa

¼ cup red rice

1¼ cups water

For the miso dressing

1 tsp miso

2 tbsp light soy sauce

2 tbsp sweet soy sauce

1 tbsp mirin

2 tbsp lemon juice

½ tsp white pepper

For the garnish

¼ cup toasted sesame seeds

2 tbsp fresh parsley, chopped

METHOD

1. Rinse and drain the chickpeas. If using dried chickpeas, pre-soak and cook in salted water for 1 hour or until soft. Rinse and drain and set aside to cool.

2. Wash, cook, drain and rinse the quinoa and red rice in a pan or rice cooker with the 1¼ cups water. Cook until soft, adding more water if necessary. Set aside to cool.

3. Wash and prepare the salad greens and tomatoes and slice the radish and silken tofu thinly.

4. Prepare the dressing by shaking all the ingredients in a jam jar or you can blend the ingredients in a small blender.

5. When you are ready to serve, place the grains on the salad leaves, tomatoes and radish and place the silken tofu on top of the grains. Pour the dressing over the tofu.

6. Garnish with freshly chopped parsley and sesame seeds and serve immediately.

CAMPUR DIPPING SALAD

KCAL 400 | PROTEIN 25g | FAT 23g | CARBS 30g | SERVES 4

INGREDIENTS

1 medium sweet potato

2 small carrots

200g semi-firm tofu

125g edamame

100g peanuts

1 cucumber

200g fried tofu

For the dipping sauce

2 tbsp sweet soy sauce

2 tbsp rice wine vinegar

1–2 red chilli peppers

METHOD

1. Peel the sweet potato and carrots and slice lengthwise. Rinse, drain and slice the semi-firm tofu. Steam sweet potato, carrots and tofu with edamame until just soft.

2. Toast the peanuts by spreading them on a baking tray and grilling for 5–10 minutes or until they start to change colour. Watch them closely as peanuts can burn quickly.

3. Wash and slice the cucumber; pat dry and set aside.

4. Prepare the dipping sauce by mixing all the ingredients together.

5. Arrange all the vegetables, peanuts and fried tofu on a serving plate and serve with the dipping sauce.

Note

1. You can use tinned edamame if you don't have fresh ones available.

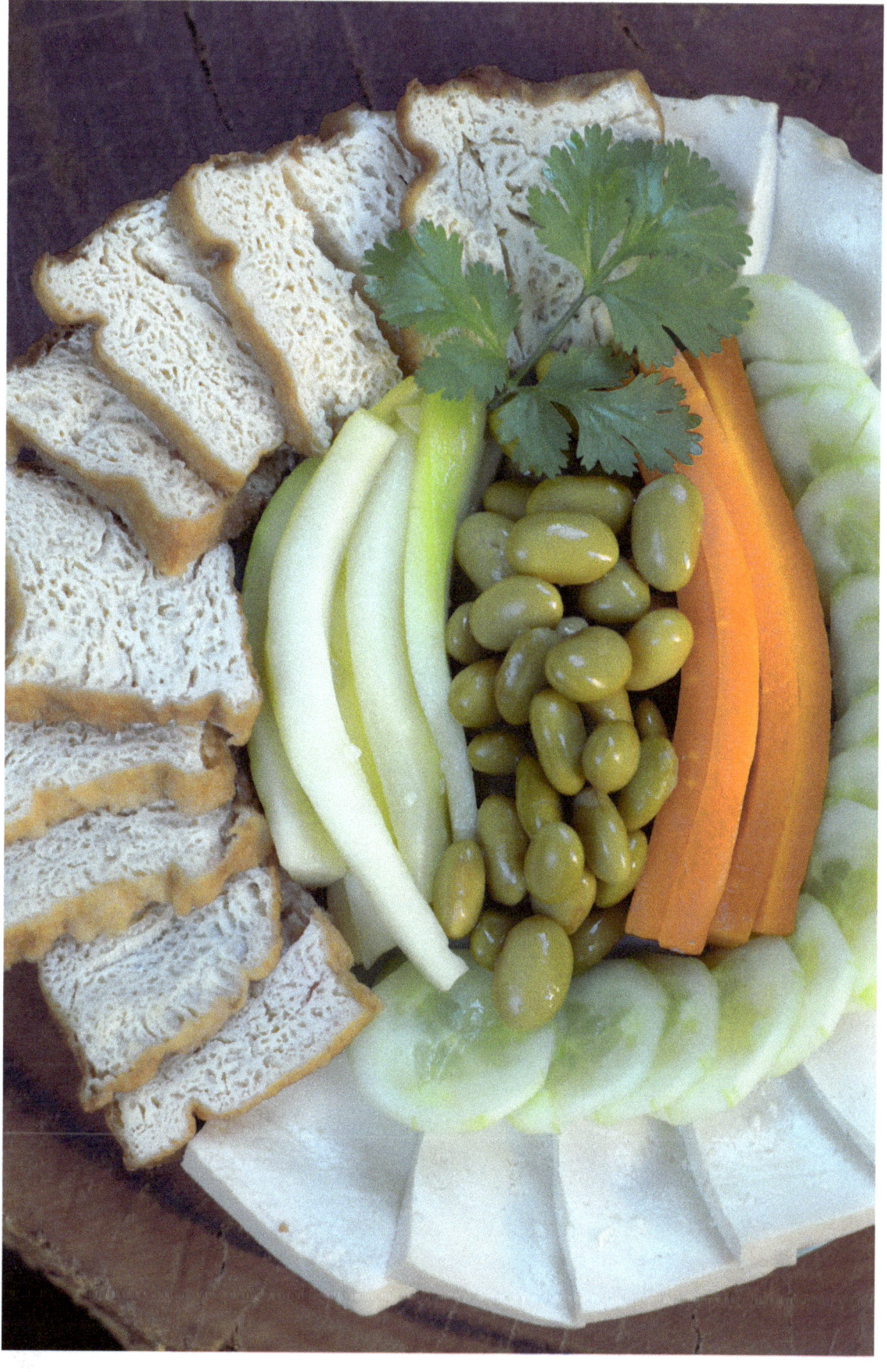

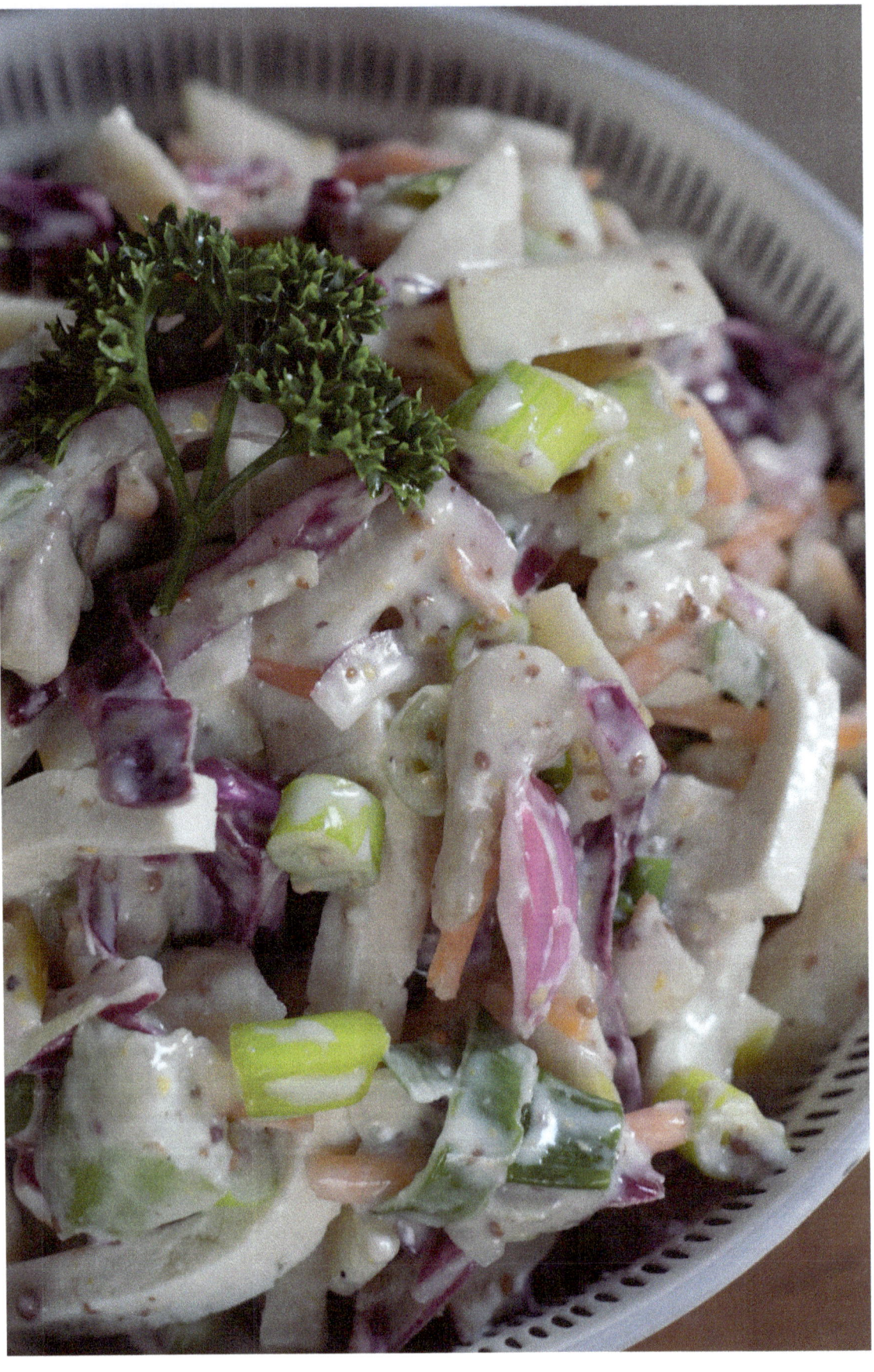

COLESLAW SALAD WITH MAYO

KCAL 198 | PROTEIN 13g | FAT 8.7g | CARBS 22g | SERVES 4

INGREDIENTS

For the salad

1 small head cabbage

1 carrot

2 red onion

5 spring onions

½ apple

300g soft tofu

For the mayonnaise

100g silken or soft tofu

1 clove garlic, peeled

1 tbsp extra-virgin olive oil

1 tsp French Dijon wholegrain mustard

1 tbsp lemon juice

1 tbsp apple cider vinegar

pinch of salt or to taste

pinch of black pepper

For the garnish

fresh parsley, chopped

METHOD

1. **For the salad** – Wash the vegetables. Shred the cabbage and carrots and thinly slice the onion, spring onions and apple.

2. Rinse and drain the tofu and cut into sticks.

3. **For the mayonnaise** – Place all the ingredients in a blender and blend until smooth.

4. Combine the salad in the mayonnaise and serve topped with fresh chopped parsley.

Notes

1. Soft or semi-firm tofu works well for this recipe.

2. If you can't source French Dijon wholegrain mustard, substitute with a different mustard.

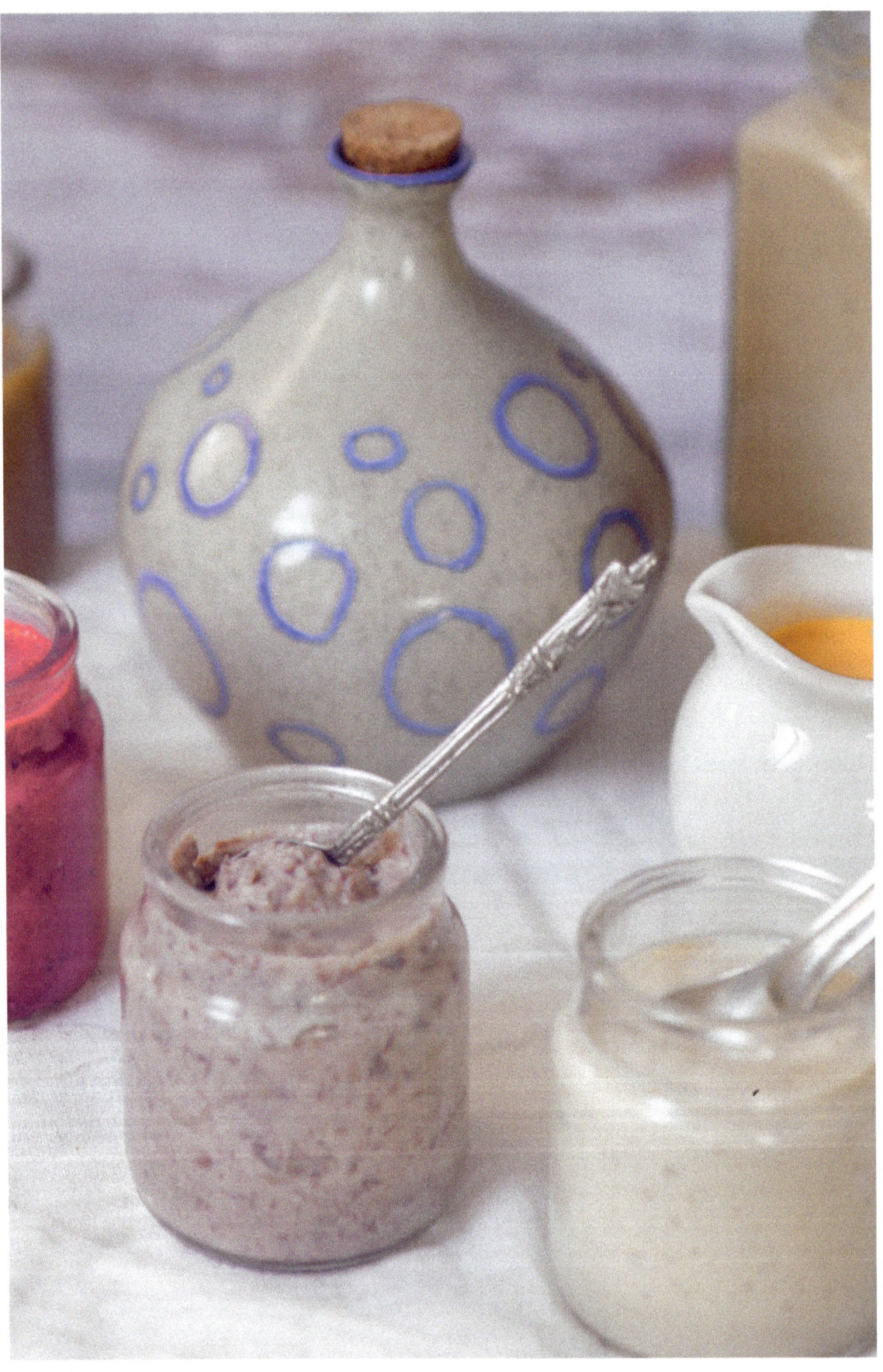

DRESSINGS

A small selection of recipes has been collated here as a 'go-to' source of inspiration for high-protein salad dressings.

Salads are healthy and nutritious, but the dressing often lets the salad down in terms of macronutrient ratios. Oil in dressings is the main culprit for raising the calories in a simple salad. This small selection offers high-protein alternatives that keep calories in check.

There are also some more ideas for dressings in the **'Salads'** chapter – for example, the *miso dressing* in the *'Quinoa and red rice salad'* on page 119 and *mayonnaise* in the *'Coleslaw salad with mayo'* on page 123. There is also a recipe for *'Creamy garlic aioli dip'* in the **'Snacks'** chapter on page 52.

FRENCH VINAIGRETTE

KCAL 118 | PROTEIN 7.4g | FAT 6.7g | CARBS 9.9g | SERVES 8

INGREDIENTS

3 tbsp extra-virgin olive oil

7 tbsp balsamic vinegar

1 tbsp French mustard

pinch of salt

12 tbsp nutritional yeast flakes

¼ cup water

METHOD

1. Place all ingredients except the water in a blender.

2. Add the water incrementally and blend until smooth. Adjust the water to achieve the desired consistency.

3. Transfer to a jar or jug to serve.

Note

1. This vinaigrette may be stored in a jar in the refrigerator for 2–4 weeks.

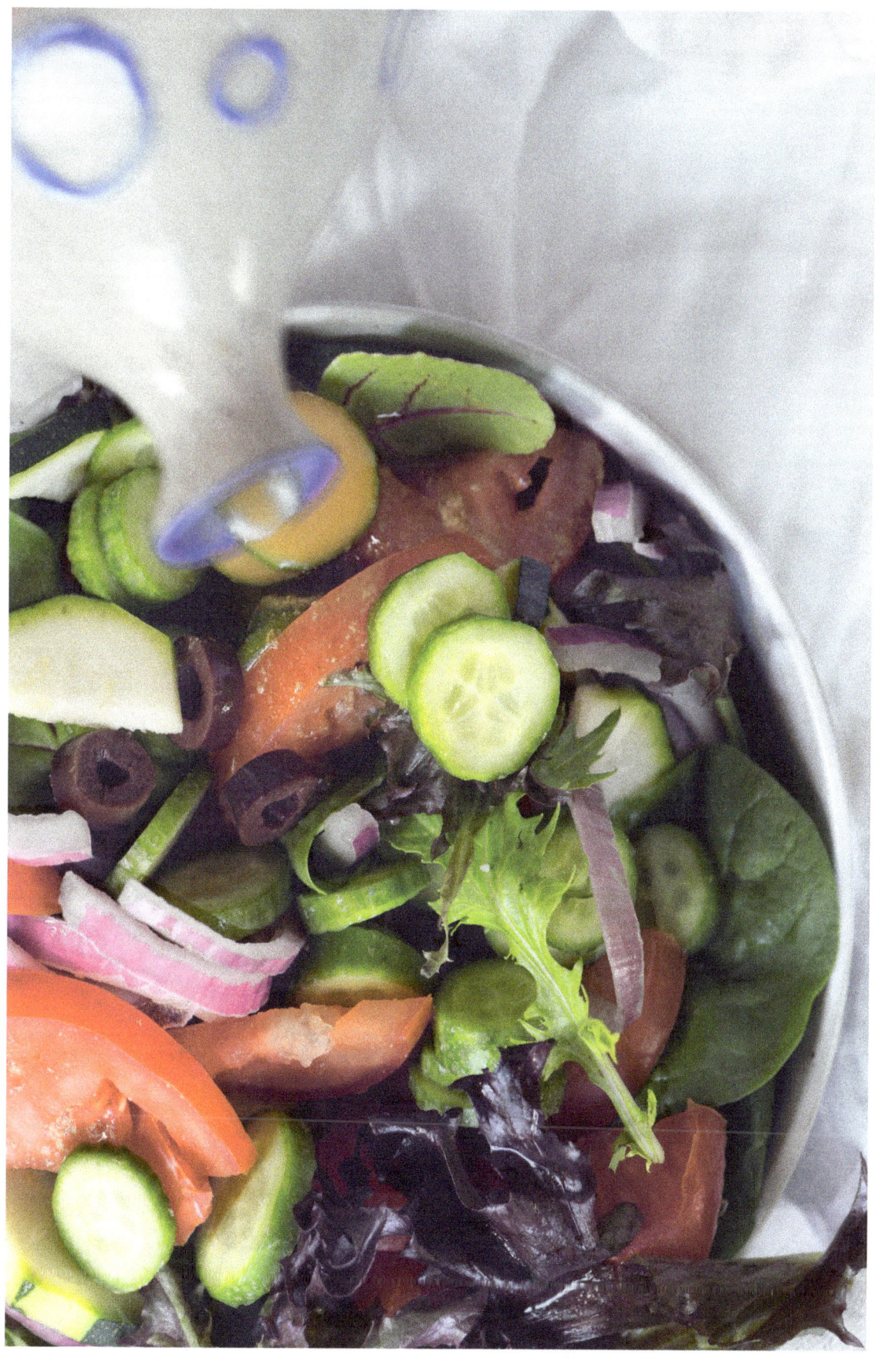

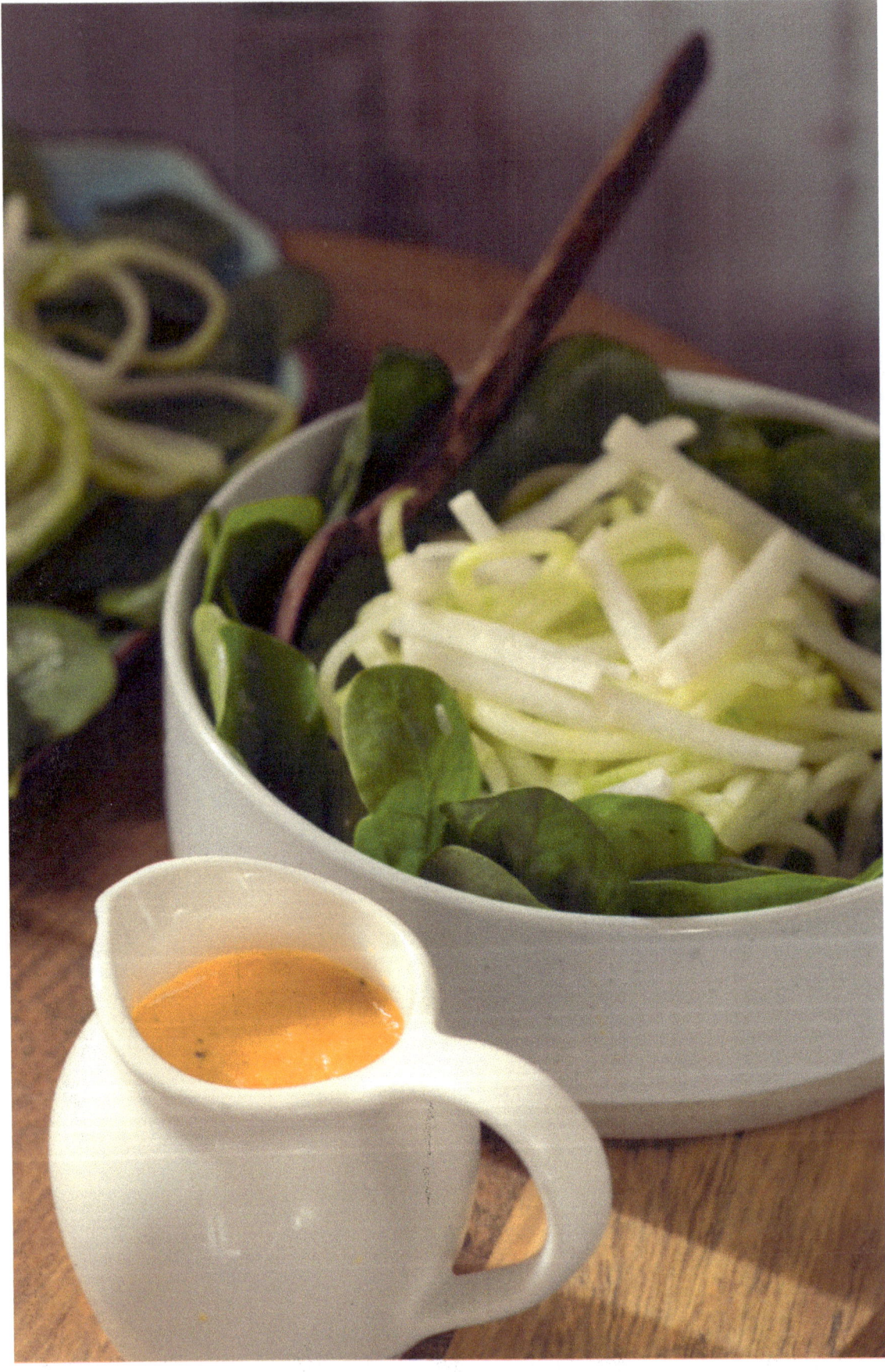

ROAST CARROT DRESSING

KCAL 81 | PROTEIN 4.3g | FAT 3.7g | CARBS 9g | SERVES 8

INGREDIENTS

500g carrots, sliced lengthwise

1 white onion, sliced

1 tbsp extra-virgin olive oil

1 tbsp Italian herbs

pinch of salt

350g soft or silken tofu

1 tsp paprika

1 tbsp lemon juice

¼ cup light soy milk

METHOD

1. Peel the carrots and onion and slice lengthwise. Place on a baking tray with a light spray of oil and sprinkle herbs and salt on top.

2. Roast in the oven on medium heat for approximately 15 minutes or until the carrots start to turn colour. Turn off the heat and cool.

3. Blend all the ingredients until smooth.

4. Transfer to a jar or jug to serve.

Note

1. This dressing can be stored in a jar in the refrigerator for 2–3 days.

LEMON CAESAR DRESSING

KCAL 26 | PROTEIN 2.8g | FAT 1.4g | CARBS 1.2g | SERVES 8

INGREDIENTS

250g soft or silken tofu

1 tsp capers

1 clove garlic, peeled

pinch of white pepper

¼ cup lemon juice

pinch of black salt or to taste

1 tsp French mustard

METHOD

1. Place all the ingredients in a blender.

2. Blend until smooth.

3. Transfer to a jar or jug to serve.

Notes

1. This dressing will keep in a jar in the refrigerator for 2–3 days.

2. Adjust seasoning to taste.

3. If you don't have black salt, substitute with regular salt.

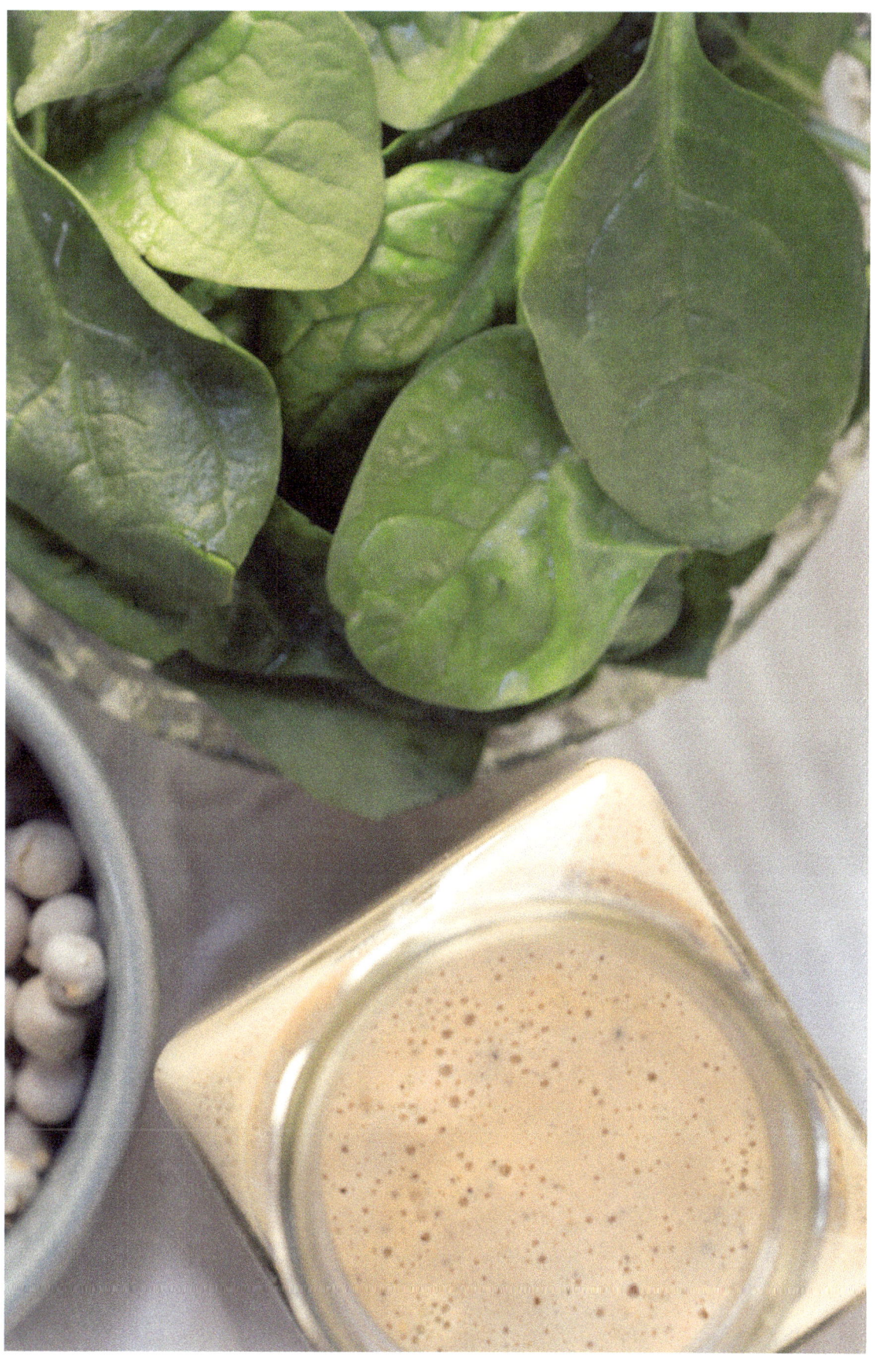

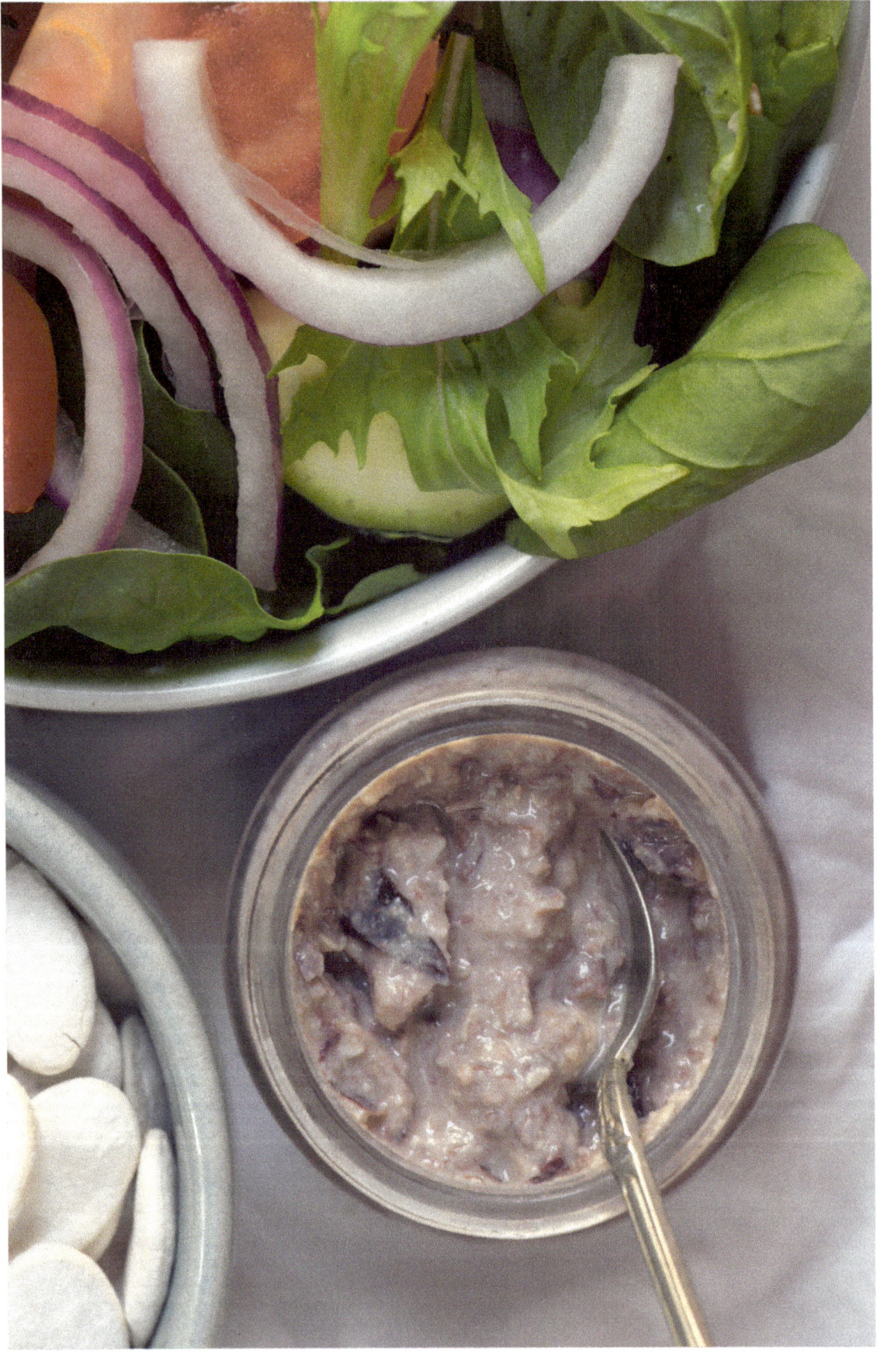

OLIVE MAYONNAISE DRESSING

KCAL 42 | PROTEIN 3.2g | FAT 2.8g | CARBS 1.9g | SERVES 8

INGREDIENTS

⅓ cup mixed olives

300g soft or silken tofu

3 cloves garlic, peeled

pinch of salt

3 tbsp lemon juice

3 tbsp capers

4 tbsp fresh parsley, chopped

3 tbsp light soy milk

METHOD

1. Drain the olives and check they are all pitted by slicing in half.

2. Place all the ingredients in a blender.

3. Blend, adjusting the quantity of soy milk to achieve the desired consistency.

4. Transfer to a jar or pot to serve.

Note

1. This dressing may be kept in a jar in the refrigerator for 2–3 days.

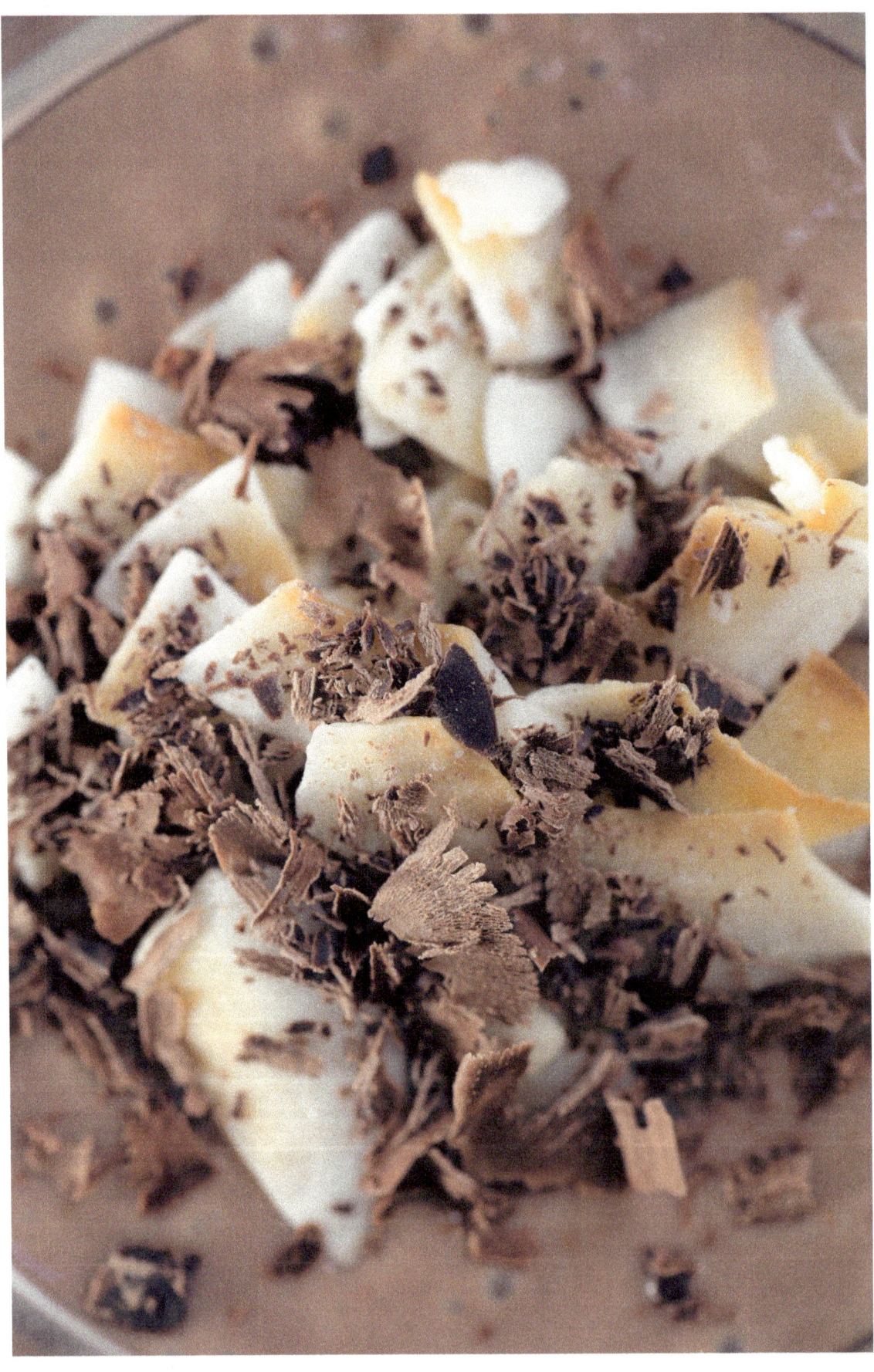

DESSERTS

Who doesn't enjoy a fresh dessert? Well, now you can without compromising your diet goals at the same time! These recipes are our high-protein dessert favourites. Some are super-fast and easy to whip up, such as the 'Choc almond dessert' and 'Strawberry mousse', whilst others take more preparation, such as the 'Choc churros'. But we promise you – they are worth it!

The 'Almond flaked rice' uses whole grain brown flaked rice available from health-food shops – well worth looking out for it as it is so delicious and filling. If you can't find brown flaked rice you can use white flaked rice. The 'Raisin and cinnamon semolina' is also a great choice for a warm dessert suited to those cooler winter days.

STRAWBERRY MOUSSE

KCAL 155 | PROTEIN 11g | FAT 8.5g | CARBS 26g | SERVES 4

INGREDIENTS

350g soft tofu
300g strawberries
4 tbsp stevia or to taste
⅛ tsp xanthan gum
4 tbsp black chia seeds

For the topping
fresh strawberries, sliced

METHOD

1. Combine all the ingredients except the chia seeds in a blender.

2. Blend until smooth, then stir in the chia seeds.

3. Transfer the mixture into serving cups. Refrigerate for at least 2 hours.

4. Top with fresh sliced strawberries and serve.

Note

1. You can easily mix in or substitute other berries of the same quantity.

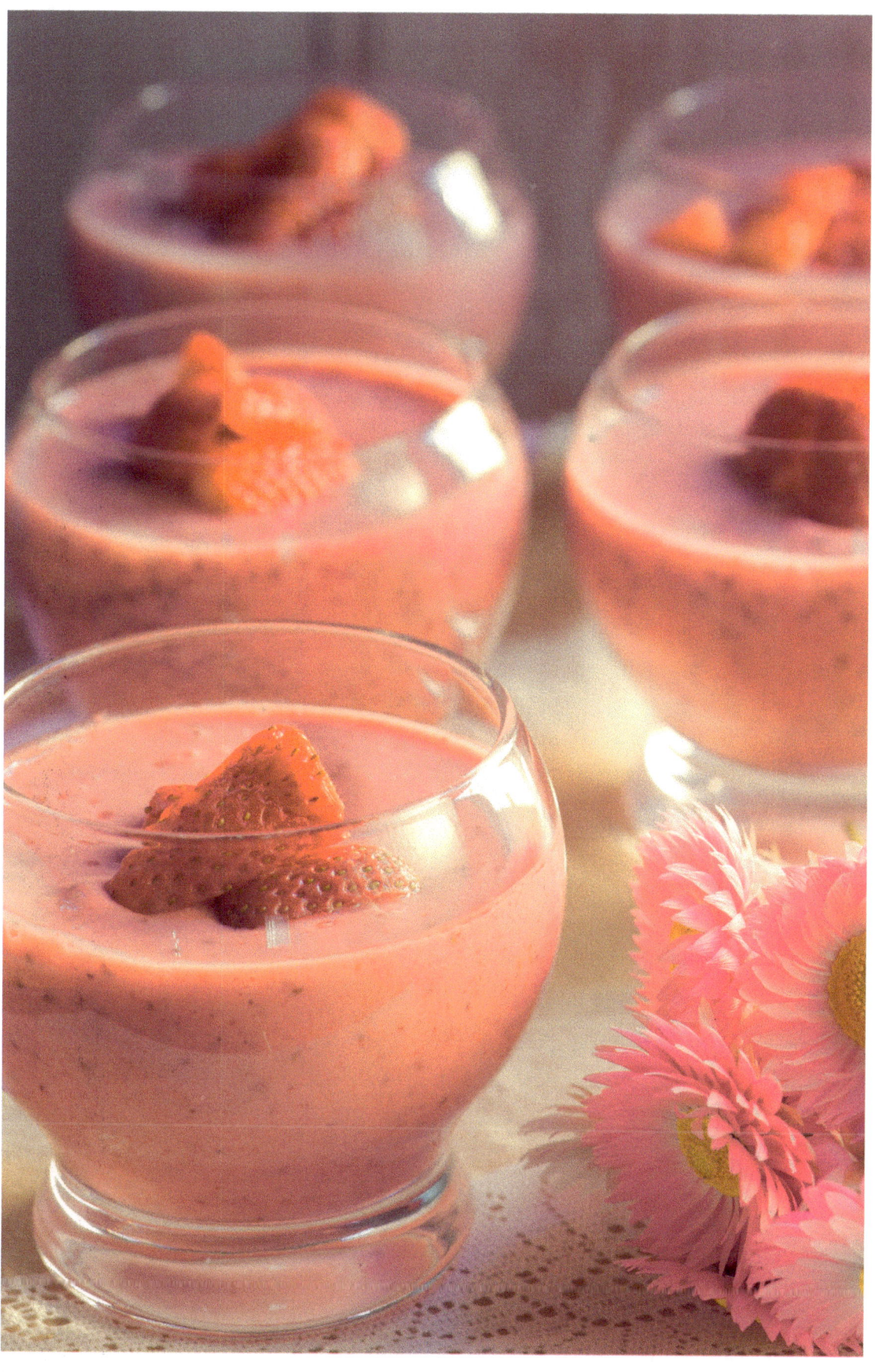

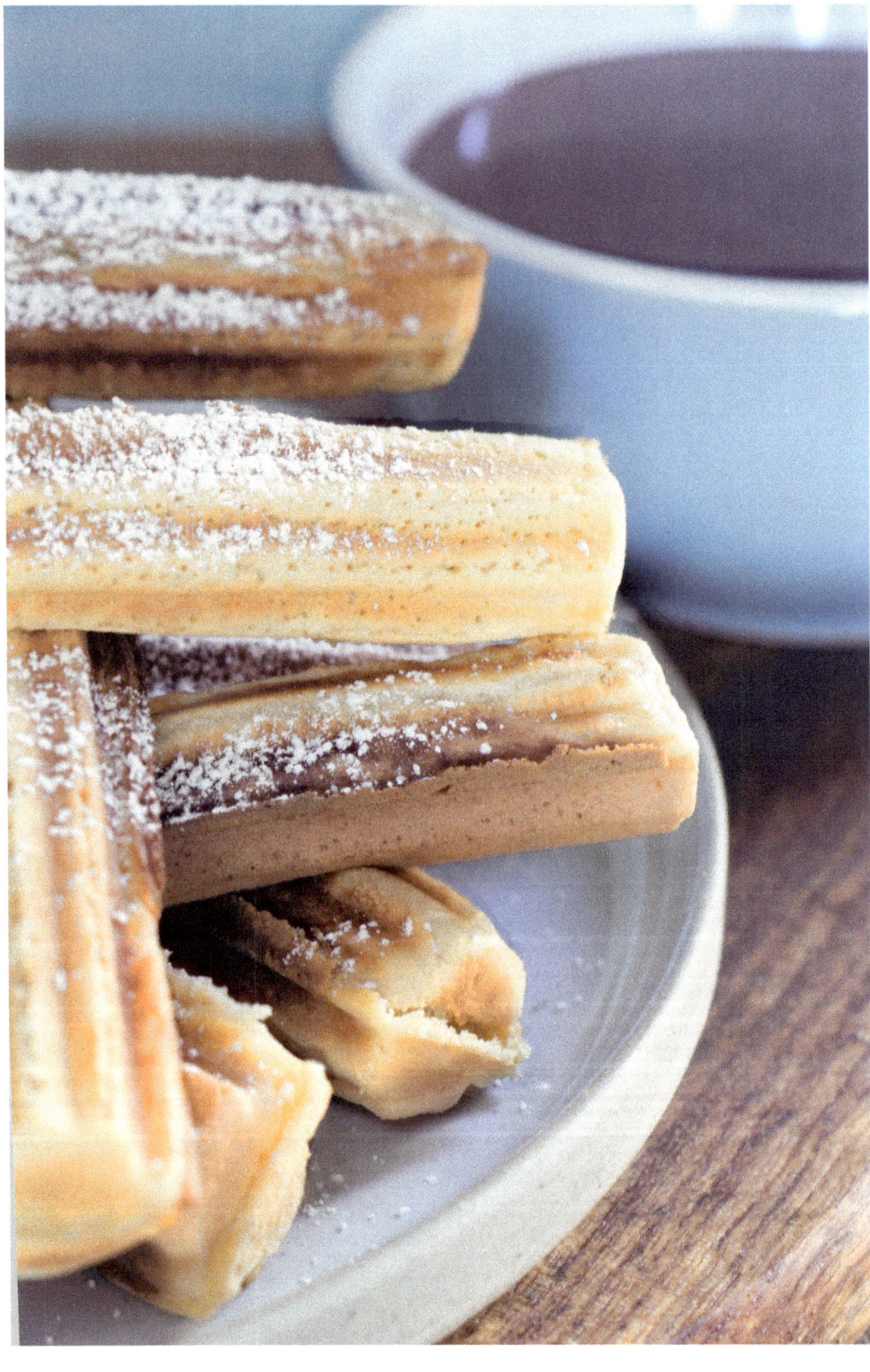

CHOC CHURROS

KCAL 248 | PROTEIN 9g | FAT 6g | CARBS 43g | SERVES 10 (2 churros per serve)

INGREDIENTS

For the churros

350g buckwheat flour

1 tsp stevia

1 tbsp flaxseed

1 tsp cinnamon

3 tsp baking powder

4 tsp cornflour

1 tsp nutmeg

pinch of salt

1½ cups light soy milk

1 tsp vanilla essence

1 tbsp coconut oil

1 tbsp lemon juice

For the chocolate sauce

2 tbsp cornflour

8 tbsp cocoa powder

4 cups light soy milk

2 tsp vanilla essence

4 tbsp stevia or to taste

To serve

coconut flour, finely ground (optional)

METHOD

1. **For the churros** – Mix the dry ingredients for the churros in a large bowl. Then add the soy milk, vanilla essence, coconut oil and lemon juice incrementally into the middle of the bowl, stirring into the dry mix to ensure there are no lumps. The mixture should be spoonable – go ahead and add more soy milk if necessary.

2. Transfer the mixture into a churros grill to cook the churros. If you don't have a churros grill you can transfer the mixture into a cake-icing bag and squeeze the mixture in lines onto a non-stick baking tray. Then bake on a medium heat for 10–15 minutes or until the churros are beginning to brown.

3. **For the chocolate sauce** – Whisk the cornflour and cocoa powder with a small amount of the soy milk until smooth with no lumps. Then transfer to a pan with the remaining soy milk, vanilla essence and stevia and heat on a medium heat, stirring until thickened.

4. Serve churros dusted with finely ground coconut flour if desired and with the chocolate sauce on the side for dipping.

ALMOND FLAKED RICE

KCAL 242 | PROTEIN 13g | FAT 4.4g | CARBS 41g | SERVES 2

INGREDIENTS

260g cooked great northern beans (or 90g dried beans)

3 cups rich soy milk

50g brown flaked rice

½ tsp cinnamon

½ tsp nutmeg

½ tsp cardamom

2 tbsp stevia or to taste

pinch of salt

1 tbsp malt extract

For the topping

10 almonds, sliced

METHOD

1. Rinse and drain the beans. If using dried beans, pre-soak, cook, rinse and drain. Combine with 1 cup of the soy milk and blend until smooth.

2. Transfer the mixture into a pan with the remaining ingredients except the malt extract. Heat on medium heat whilst stirring.

3. When warm, stir in the malt extract. Continue stirring until the dessert has thickened.

4. Transfer the dessert to serving bowls and garnish with the sliced almonds to serve.

Notes

1. You can buy white or brown flaked rice from health-food stores. This recipe assumes you are using brown flaked rice but you can also use white.

2. You can use white beans or cannelloni beans in place of great northern beans.

3. You can make 'rich' soy milk by following the instructions in the recipe for 'Home-made soy milk blend' on page 158, or go ahead and use store-purchased soy milk.

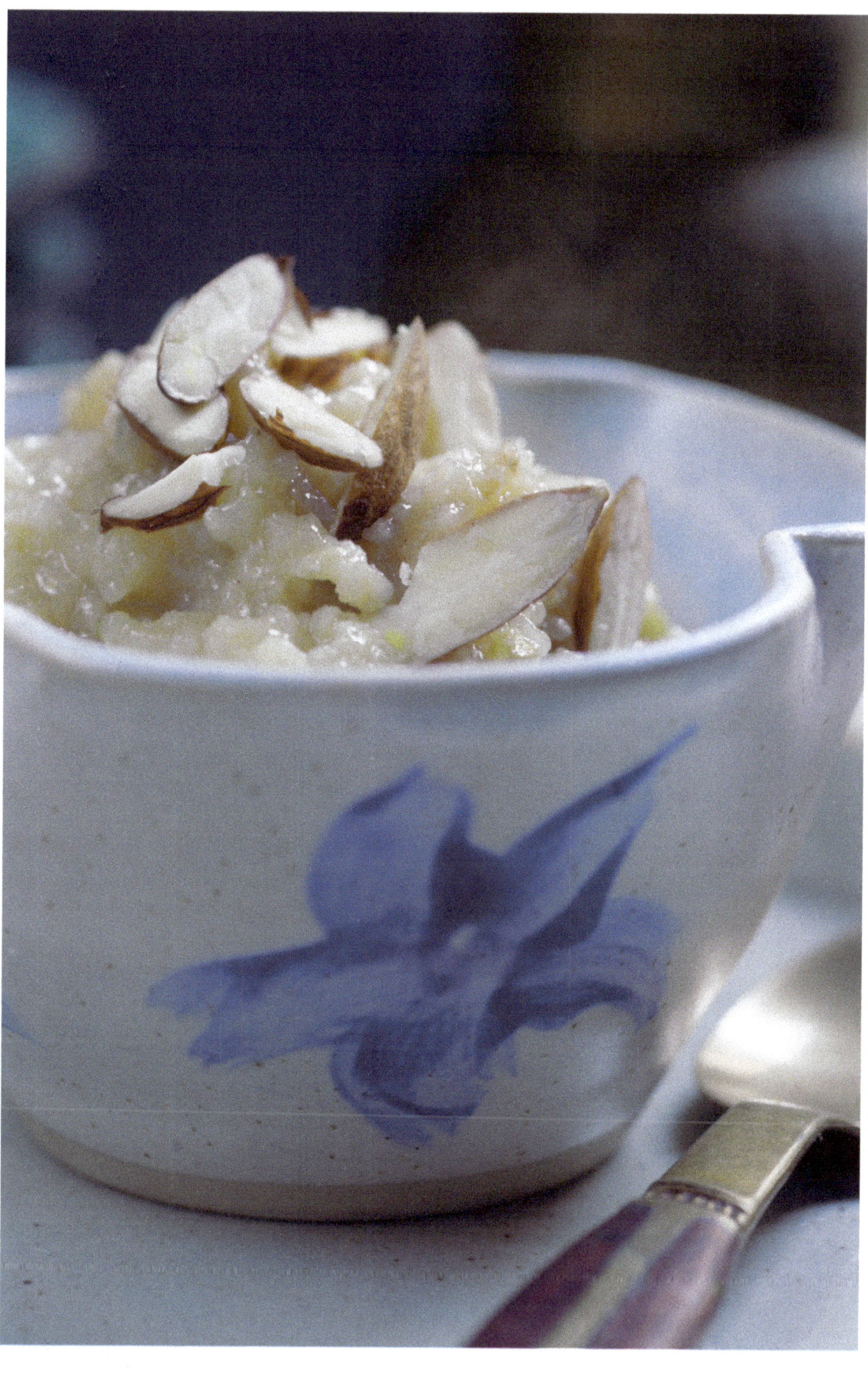

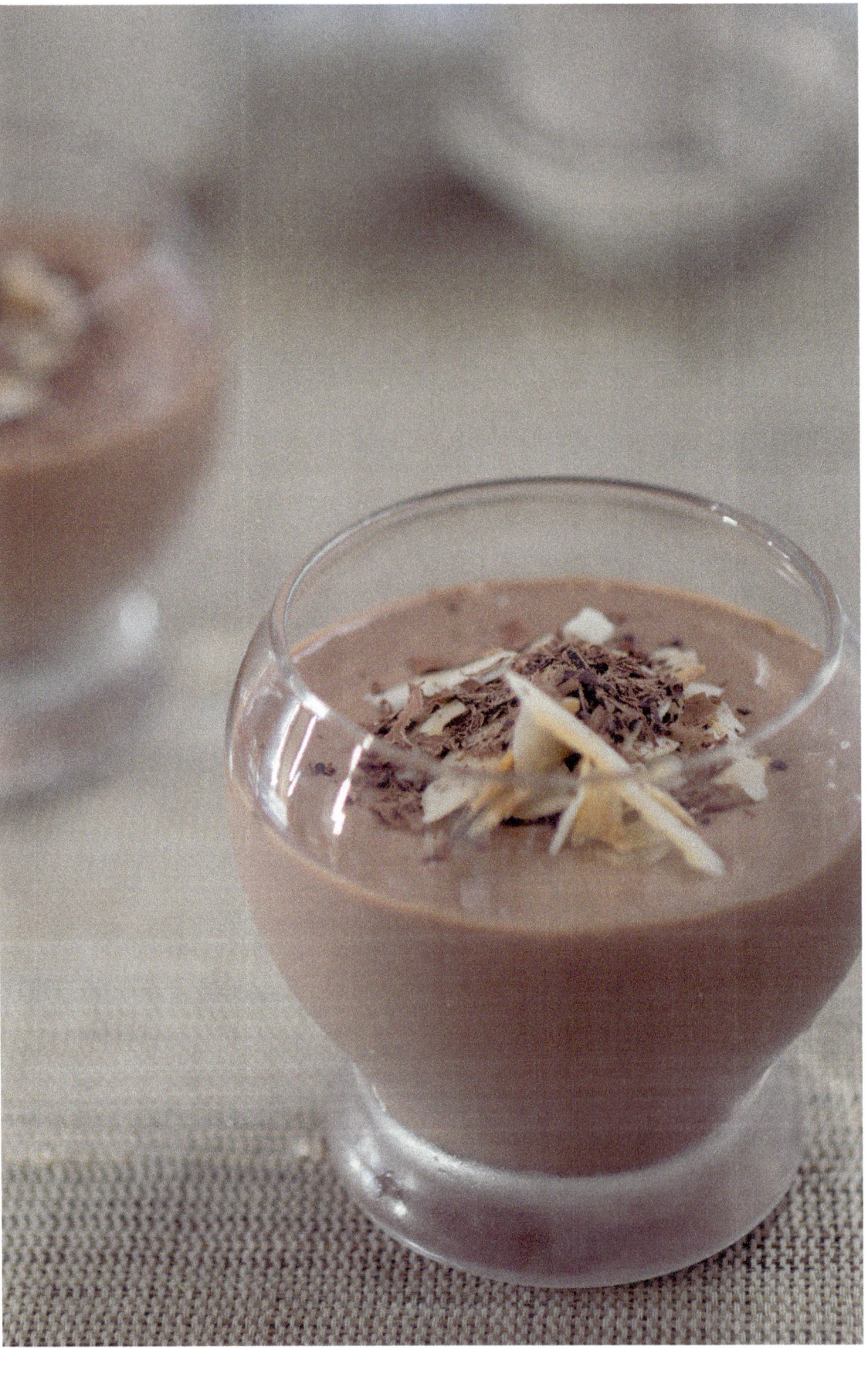

CHOC ALMOND DESSERT

KCAL 347 | PROTEIN 23g | FAT 19g | CARBS 41g | SERVES 2

INGREDIENTS

300g soft tofu

6 heaped tsp cocoa powder

6 tsp stevia

⅛ tsp xanthan gum

20 almonds

4 dates

200ml light soy milk

For the topping

10g dark vegan chocolate, shaved

1 tsp cocoa nibs

1 tbsp coconut flakes

METHOD

1. Place all the ingredients except the soy milk into a blender. Add the soy milk incrementally and blend until the mixture is smooth and of the desired consistency.

2. Pour mixture into serving bowls and refrigerate to set.

3. Top with shaved dark chocolate, cocoa nibs and coconut flakes to serve.

Note

1. The end consistency of this dessert depends in part on the type of tofu you use. Soft tofu is likely to result in a firmer dessert. If you use a silken tofu, use less soy milk to achieve your preferred consistency.

RAISIN & CINNAMON SEMOLINA

KCAL 218 | PROTEIN 12g | FAT 2.5g | CARBS 43g | SERVES 4

INGREDIENTS

350g cooked great northern beans (or 120g dried beans)

2 cups light soy milk

¼ cup semolina

2 tbsp stevia or to taste

½ tsp cinnamon

½ tsp nutmeg

½ tsp cardamom

1 tsp malt extract

¼ cup raisins

For the topping

cinnamon powder

METHOD

1. Rinse and drain the beans. If using dried beans, pre-soak, cook, rinse and drain. Combine with the soy milk and blend until very smooth.

2. Transfer the mixture into a pan with the remaining ingredients except the malt extract and raisins. Heat on medium heat, stirring.

3. When warm, stir in the malt extract and raisins. Continue stirring until the mixture thickens.

4. Transfer into serving dishes and sprinkle with cinnamon to serve.

Note

1. You can use white beans or cannelloni beans in place of great northern beans.

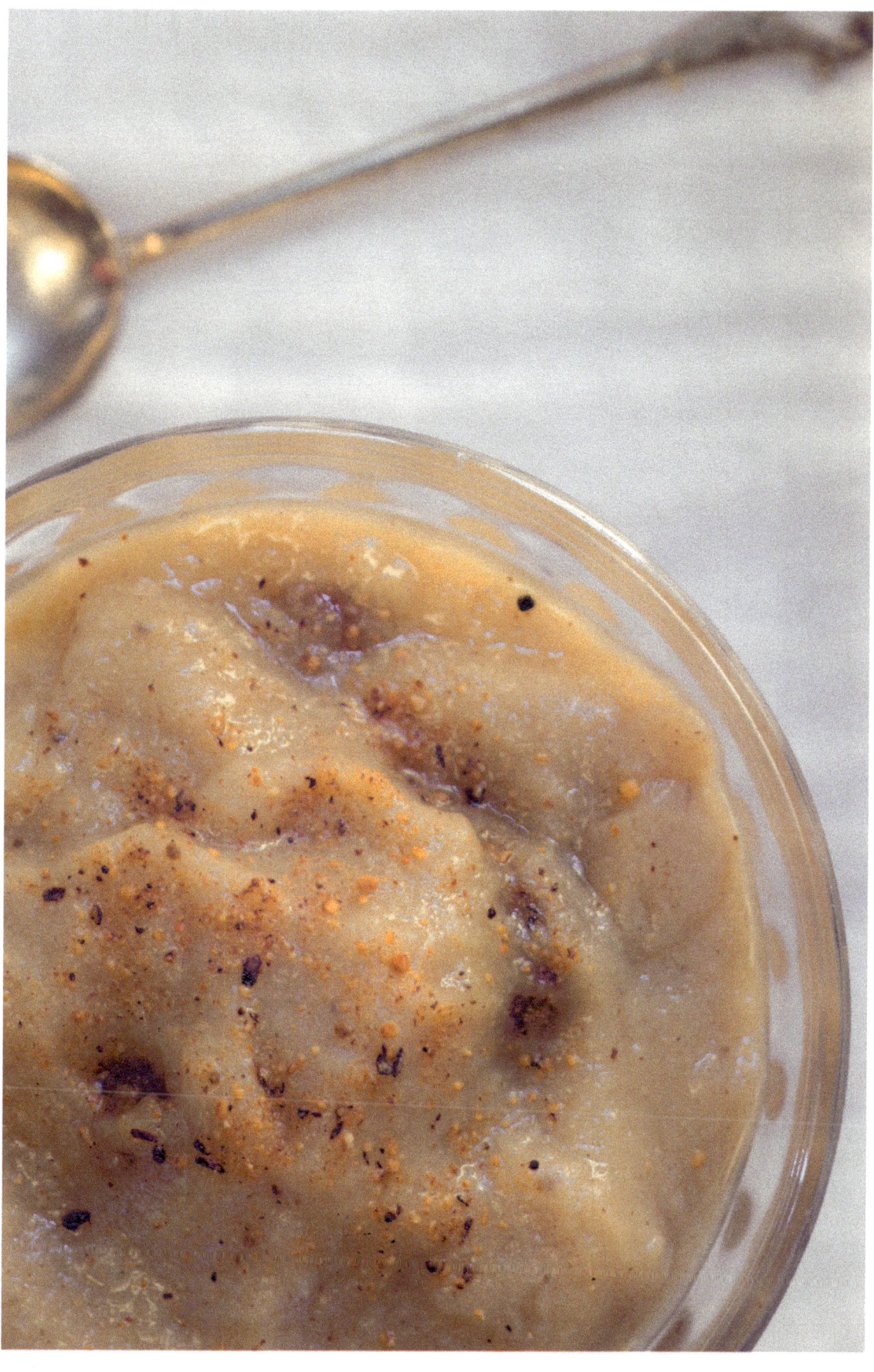

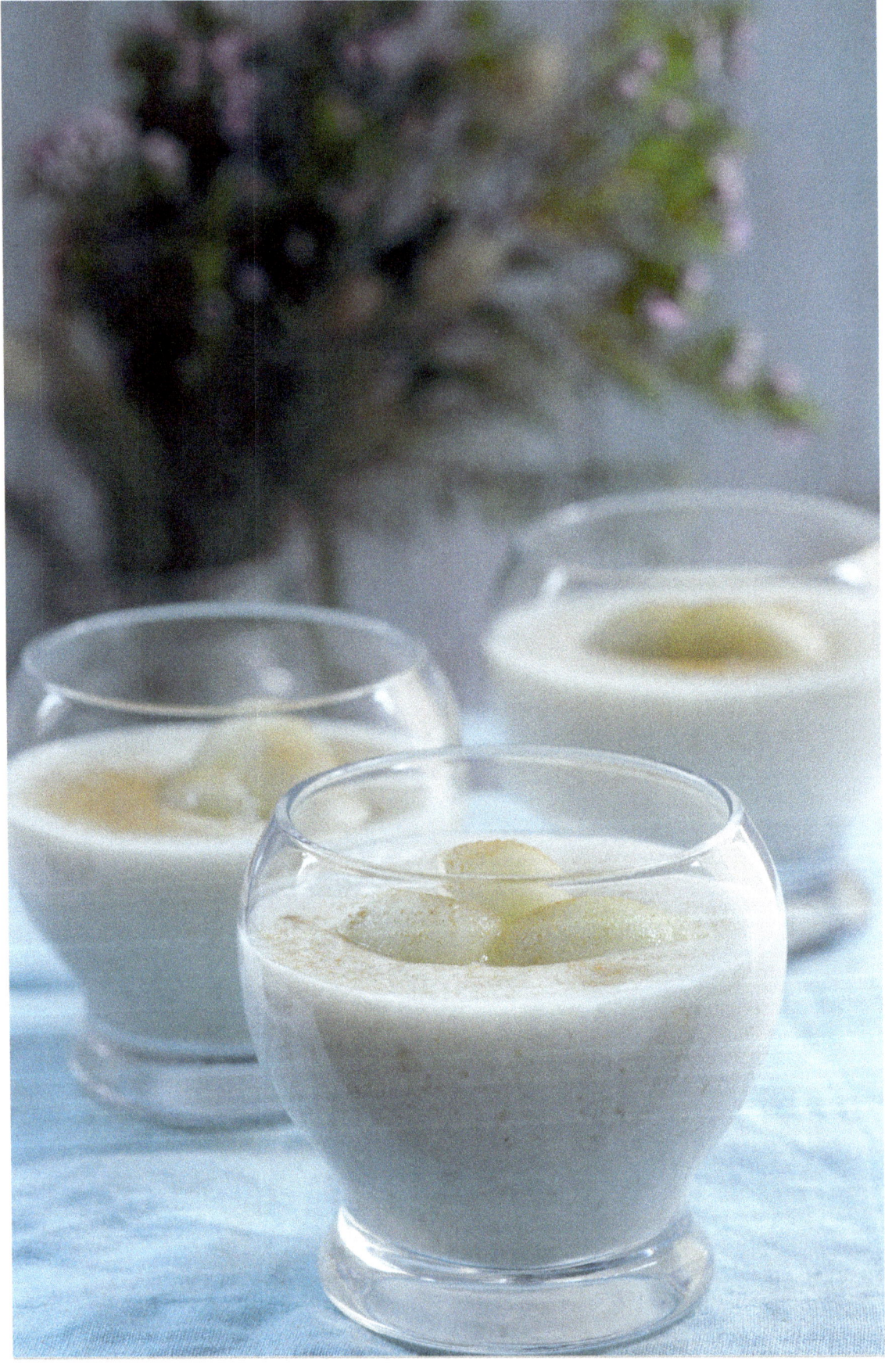

MELON COCONUT DREAM DESSERT

KCAL 97 | PROTEIN 5.8g | FAT 4.4g | CARBS 9.6g | SERVES 4

INGREDIENTS

300g soft tofu

1 tsp vanilla extract

2 cups melon balls or cubes

3 tbsp stevia or to taste

2 tbsp coconut cream

⅛ tsp xanthan gum

⅛ tsp ginger powder

For the topping

melon balls or cubes

¼ tsp ginger powder

METHOD

1. Combine all ingredients in a blender, retaining some melon for the topping. Blend until smooth.

2. Transfer mixture into serving bowls. Refrigerate for at least 2 hours.

3. Top with melon and sprinkle ginger powder over the top using a sieve to serve.

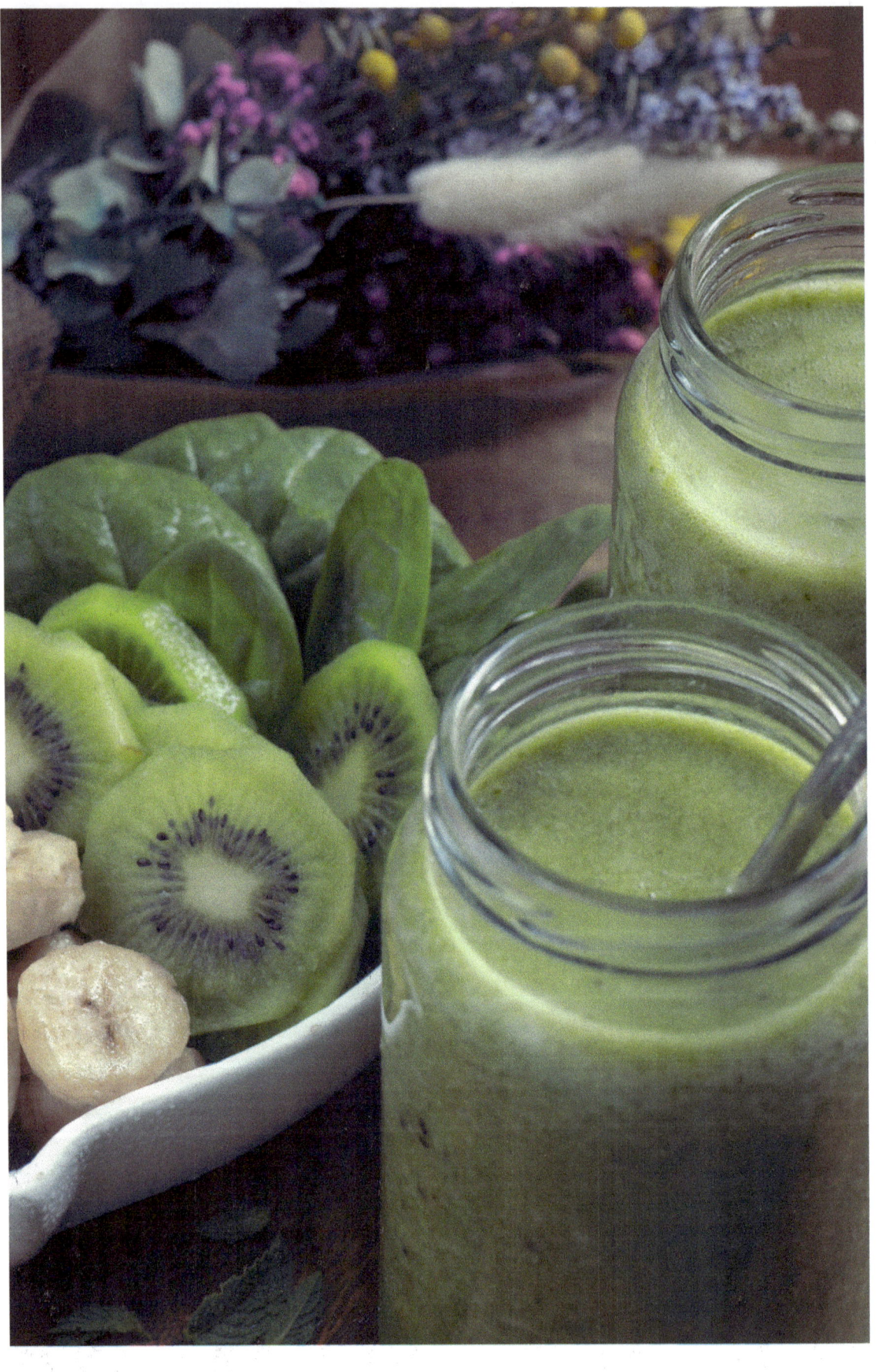

DRINKS

Perhaps surprisingly, all these drinks are 'high-protein', that is 20% or more of their calories come from protein. One of our favourites is the refreshing *Spinach smoothie*, which provides a high-protein content and superb micronutrient profile from the green goodness in this drink. It is also highly nutritious as the fruit and veggies are consumed in their raw form.

'Turmeric latte' is also one of our favourites as a warm drink in winter. The benefits of curcumin, found in turmeric, are widely documented and include its anti-inflammatory and antioxidant properties. It is important to include the black pepper as it contains piperine that helps the body to absorb the curcumin from the turmeric.

'Seasonal coconut and almond oat smoothie' is a favourite of ours that we make nearly every day. We love the blueberry version, but you can swap out the blueberries with local fruits that are in season. This smoothie base provides a combination of micronutrients essential to a good vegan diet as well as being high-protein and filling.

'Home-made soy milk blend' is another staple of ours – we prepare our soy milk fresh daily using a consumer-grade soy milk maker. By using this recipe you will gain a variety of micronutrients from the nuts and seeds as well as the soybeans.

Finally, *'Chai latte'* contains spices to aid digestion and general wellness of the body. Enjoy!

SEASONAL COCONUT & ALMOND OAT SMOOTHIE (BLUEBERRY)

KCAL 160 | PROTEIN 9.2g | FAT 7.7g | CARBS 20g | SERVES 2

INGREDIENTS

2 tbsp rolled oats

2 tsp ground almonds

2 tsp ground flaxseed

2 tsp desiccated coconut

2 cups light soy milk

80g fresh blueberries

METHOD

1. Measure out the ingredients into a blender.

2. Blend until smooth and serve.

Notes

1. You can substitute blueberries with other seasonal and local fruits.

Ripe banana or pineapple are natural choices to sweeten this smoothie – but these fruits contain higher quantities of sugar so be sure to account for this if you are counting calories.

2. You can opt to blend half the ingredients with the soy milk and then stir in the remaining half so that you have a variety of textures in the smoothie.

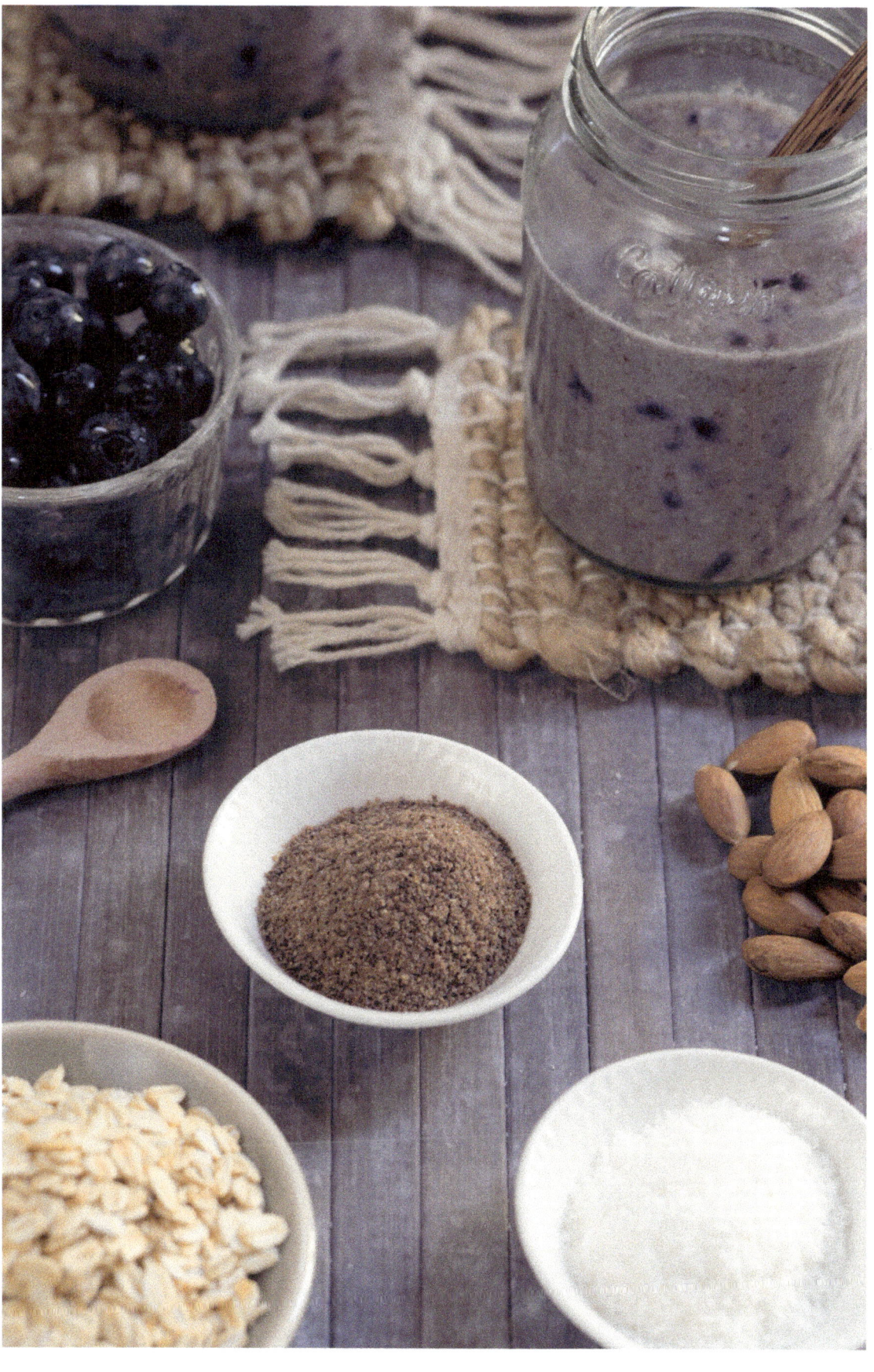

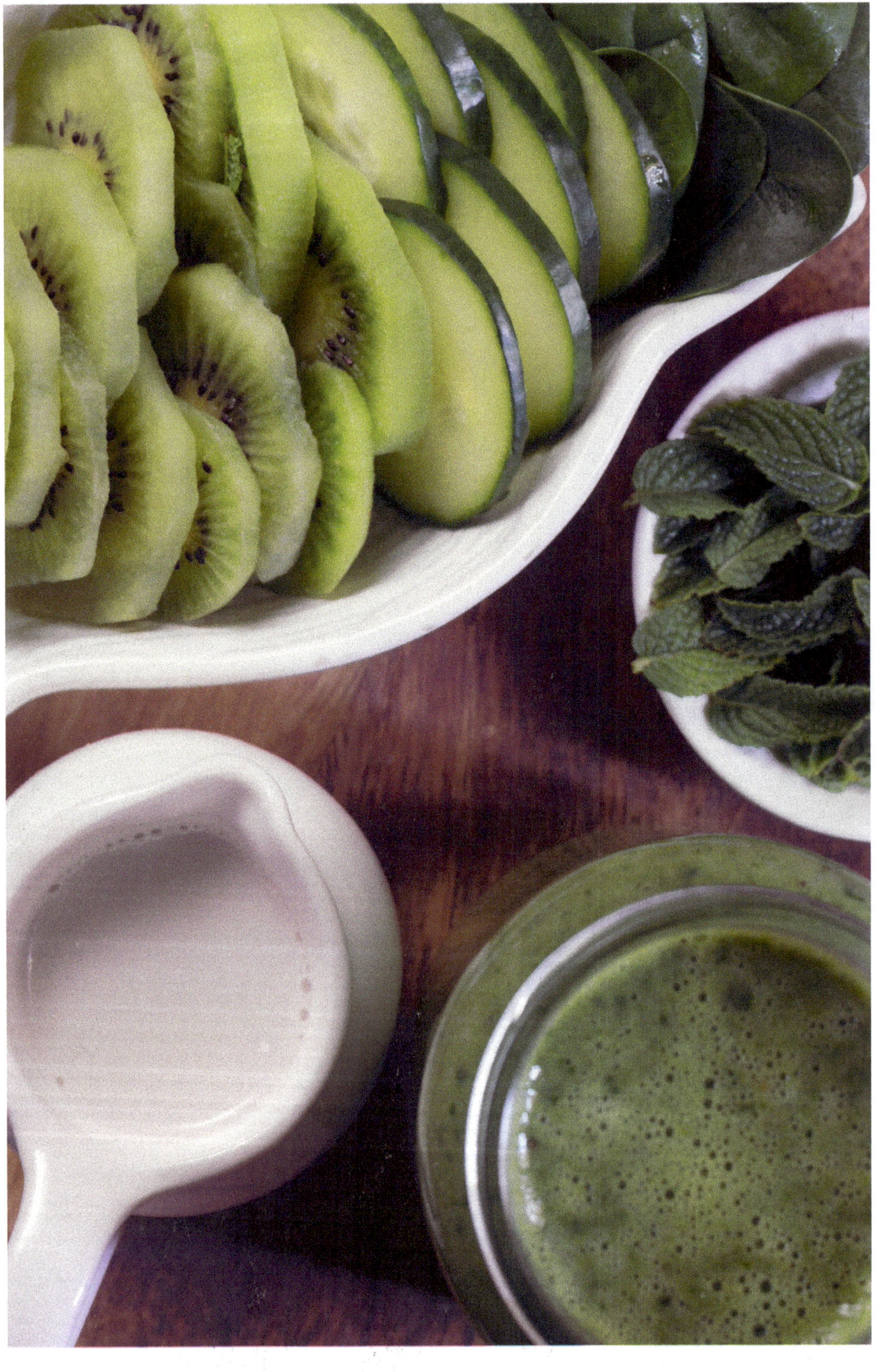

GREEN SMOOTHIE

KCAL 166 | PROTEIN 9.9g | FAT 4.7g | CARBS 27g | SERVES 2

INGREDIENTS

100g fresh spinach

½ stick celery

5 tbsp fresh mint

¼ medium cucumber, chilled

2 green kiwi fruit

1-inch stick ginger, peeled

2 cups light soy milk

1 cup water

2 tsp stevia (optional)

pinch of salt

METHOD

1. Wash the spinach, celery and mint thoroughly and drain. Peel and roughly chop the cucumber, kiwi fruit and ginger.

2. Combine all the ingredients in a blender, saving some of the fresh mint. Blend until smooth.

3. Serve immediately with fresh mint garnish.

Notes

1. You can add a cup of unsweetened coconut water, a cup of chopped pineapple, or another fruit of your choice in place of the stevia.

2. You can include 'mix-ins' such as figs, berries and seeds. Remember to update the nutritional information if you are counting calories.

TURMERIC LATTE

KCAL 154 | PROTEIN 15g | FAT 8.4g | CARBS 43g | SERVES 2

INGREDIENTS

2 cups light soy milk

pinch of black pepper

2 tsp fresh turmeric, finely chopped

4 dates

1-inch stick ginger, peeled

pinch of cinnamon

½ tsp vanilla essence

stevia to taste

METHOD

1. Blend all the ingredients until smooth.

2. Heat and bring to a boil then simmer for 2–3 minutes.

3. Strain the mixture into cups or glasses and serve.

Notes

1. This recipe is especially delicious made with the 'Homemade soy milk blend' on page 158.

2. You can make this extra frothy using a hand-held milk frother.

3. You can substitute fresh ginger with ¼ tsp ginger powder.

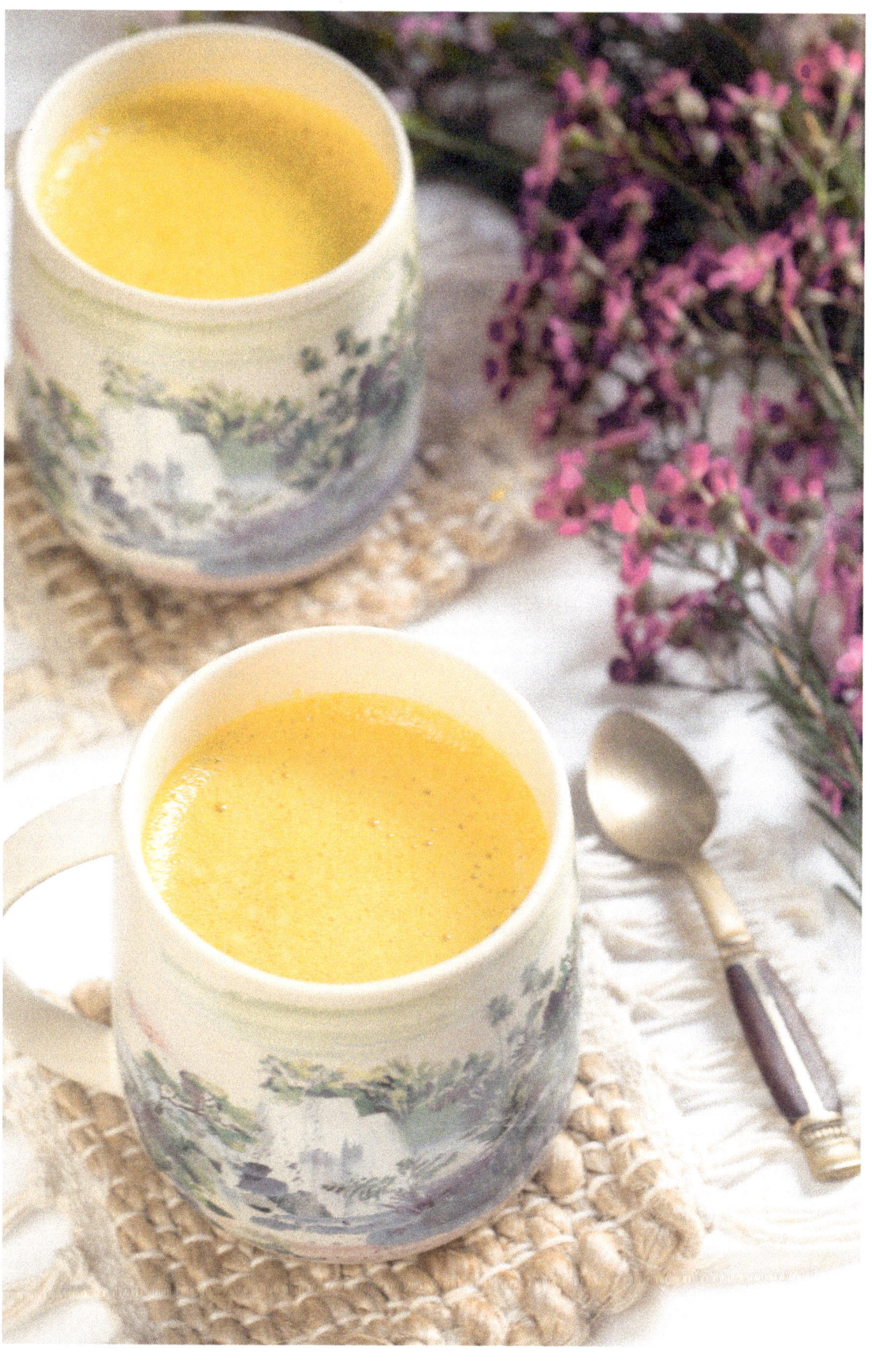

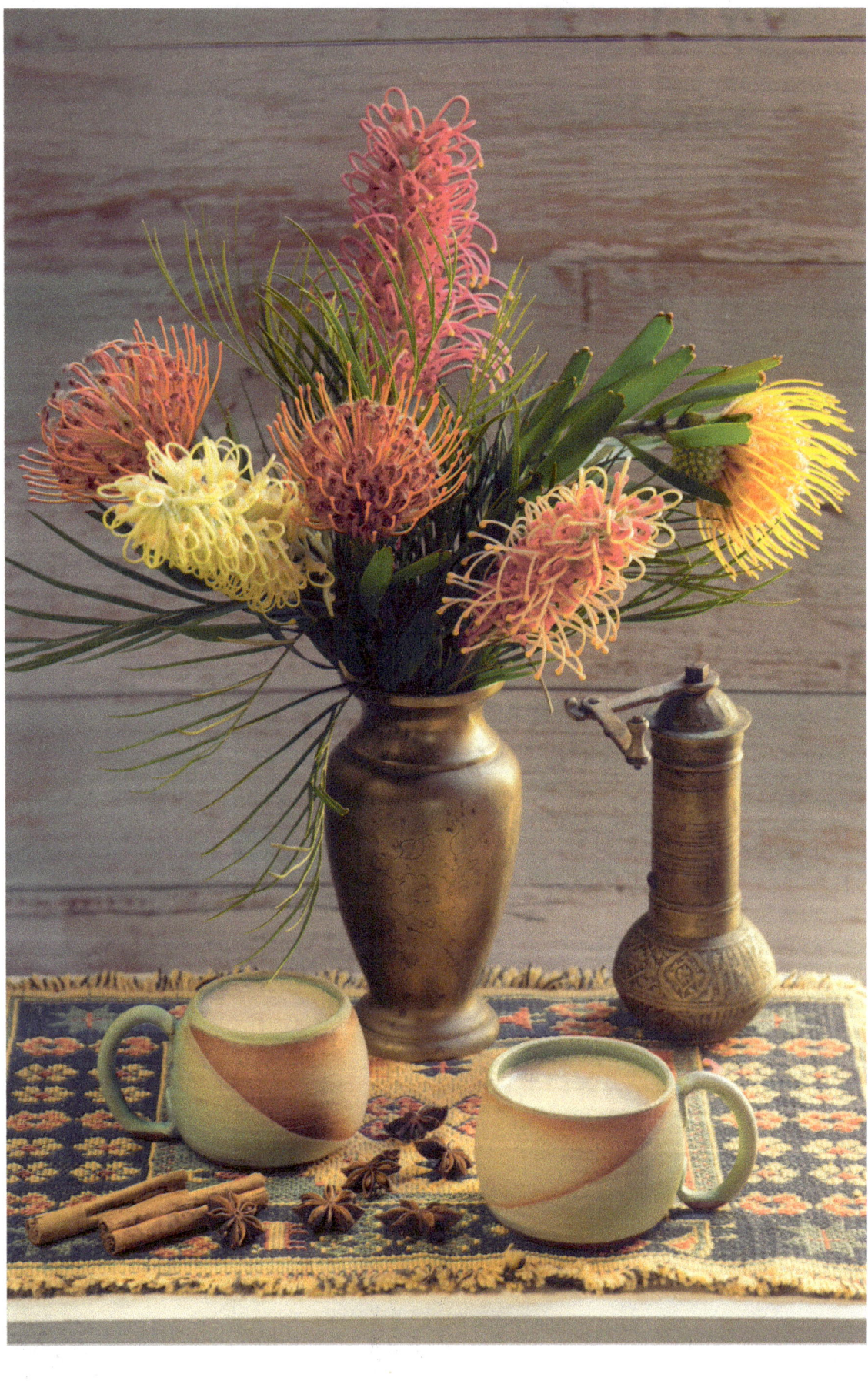

CHAI LATTE

KCAL 126 | PROTEIN 7.8g | FAT 5.1g | CARBS 13g | SERVES 2

INGREDIENTS

2 cups soy milk

2 pinches nutmeg

2 pinches black pepper

2 pinches cardamom

6 cloves

2-inch stick ginger, peeled

stevia to taste

2 tsp fresh tea leaves

To garnish

cinnamon powder

METHOD

1. Blend all the ingredients except the tea leaves and cinnamon.

2. Place the blended mix and tea leaves in a pan, bring to a boil then simmer for 2–3 minutes.

3. Strain the mixture into cups or glasses.

4. Sprinkle with cinnamon to serve.

Notes

1. This is especially delicious made with the *'Home-made soy milk blend'* on page 158.

2. You can make this extra frothy using a hand-held milk frother.

3. You can substitute fresh ginger for ¼ tsp ginger powder.

HOME MADE SOY MILK BLEND

KCAL 100 | PROTEIN 6.5g | FAT 5.2g | CARBS 6.9g | SERVES 4

INGREDIENTS

⅓ cup dried soybeans (½ cup for 'rich soy milk').

1 tbsp almonds

1 tbsp sunflower kernels

pinch of salt

1 date

½ tsp vanilla essence

4 cups water

METHOD

If you have a soy milk maker, combine all the ingredients and follow the instructions on your machine. If you don't have a maker follow the directions below.

1. Pre-soak the soybeans, almonds and sunflower kernels for 6–8 hours or overnight.

2. Drain and rinse the soybeans, almonds and sunflower kernels. Combine in a blender with the remaining ingredients. Blend until smooth. (Make sure you have a blender that is powerful enough to blend soybeans and nuts.)

3. Transfer the mixture into a pan or rice cooker and bring to the boil. Simmer for 1–1½ hours whilst monitoring consistently. Scoop off and discard the froth that forms on the top from time to time.

4. Let it cool and when warm strain into a vessel using a fine sieve. Discard the pulp (called 'okara' – see note 3) and retain the liquid milk.

Notes

1. This recipe is much easier with a consumer-grade soy milk maker.

2. To increase the richness of the milk use ½ cup dried soybeans (136 kcal, 9.4g protein, 6.8g fat, 9.2g carbohydrate).

3. The okara can be used as an ingredient in other recipes.

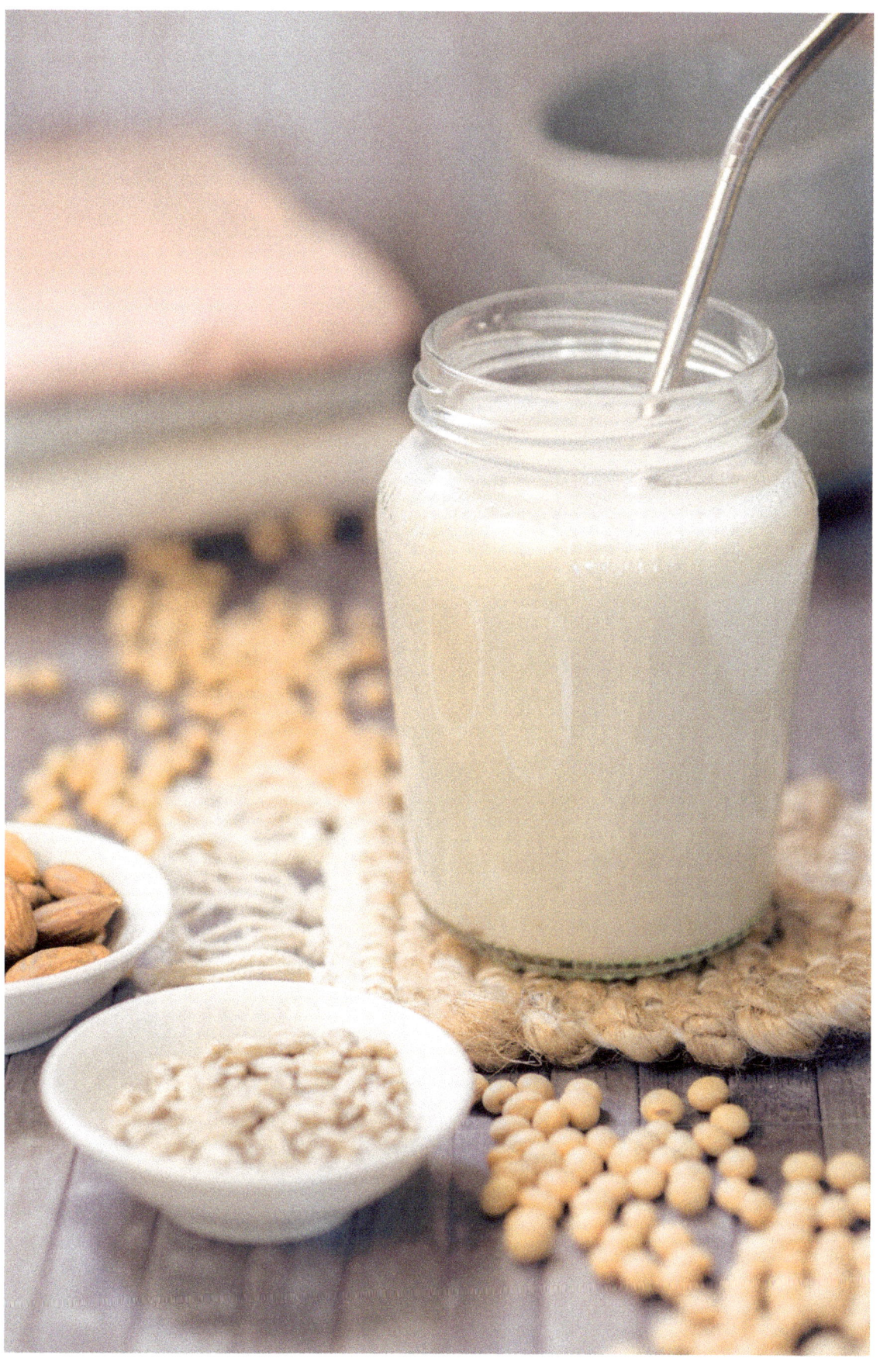

RESOURCES

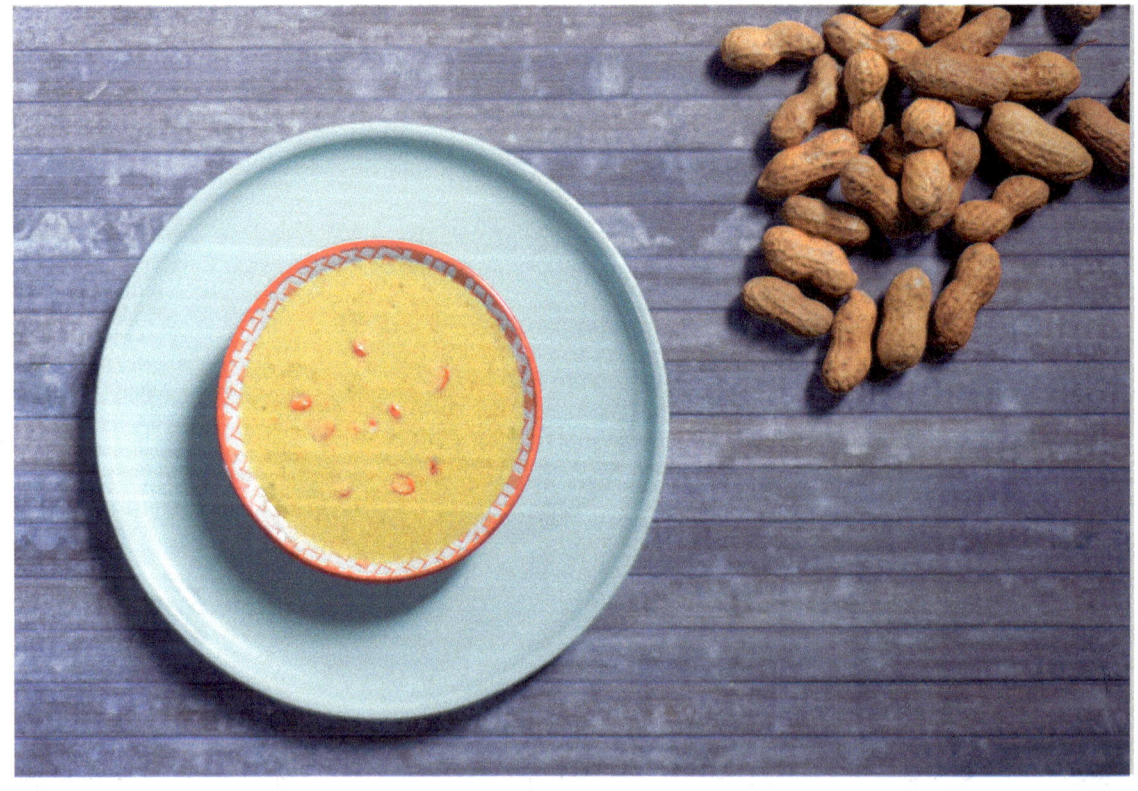

Conversion charts

OVEN M

	°C	°F	Gas mark
Low	150	300	2
Medium	180	350	4
High	200	400	6

DRY INGREDIENTS

Metric	Imperial
15g	½ oz
30g	1 oz
45g	1½ oz
60g	2 oz
75g	2½ oz
100g	3½ oz
155g	5 oz
185g	6 oz
200g	6½ oz
250g	8 oz
300g	9½ oz
350g	11 oz
375g	12 oz
400g	12½ oz
425g	13½ oz
440g	14 oz
470g	15 oz
500g	1 lb (16 oz)
750g	1 lb 0 oz
1kg (1000g)	2 lb

CUPS AND SPOONS

Cups	Metric	Imperial
1 cup	250ml	8 fl oz
½ cup	125ml	4 fl oz
¼ cup	60ml	2 fl oz

Spoons	Metric
1 tablespoon (tbsp)	20ml
1 teaspoon (tsp)	5ml
½ teaspoon (tsp)	2.5ml
¼ teaspoon (tsp)	1.25ml

LIQUID INGREDIENTS

Metric	Imperial
30ml	1 fl oz
60ml	2 fl oz
100ml	3½ fl oz
125ml	4 fl oz (½ cup)
155ml	5 fl oz
170ml	5½ fl oz
200ml	6½ fl oz
250ml	8 fl oz (1 cup)
300ml	9½ fl oz
370ml	12 fl oz
410ml	13 fl oz
470ml	15 fl oz
500ml	16 fl oz (2 cups)
600ml	1 pt (20 fl oz)
750ml	1 pt 5 fl oz
1 litre	1 pt 12 fl oz

NOTES

1. The recipes in this book are considered by Anise & Green to be vegan friendly and planet friendly. Many are also gluten free and nut free as well. However, these qualities depend on the actual ingredients you use and the environment in which you make them. As product availability varies according to where you live in the world, we have not listed specific brands of food. To ensure your ingredients are vegan and planet friendly as well as meeting the needs of your dietary requirements you must read the product labels.

2. The **nutritional information** provided is approximate and will vary according to your measurements, vessels, brands of products, appliances and other equipment, cooking style and food storage system. Nutritional information has been calculated using online calculators and provided for your convenience. We have gone to great efforts to ensure the information is as accurate as possible but can provide no warranties for its accuracy. We encourage you to make your own calculations based on the actual ingredients you use and using your own preferred nutrition calculator.

The authors are not dieticians or nutritionists. The information shared in this book is based on personal experience and research but must not be taken as medical or nutritional advice. Please consult your healthcare provider for nutritional and medical advice.

3. **Health and safety.** When using mushrooms, please refrain from picking them outside without consulting an appropriate guide for ensuring their edibility. When storing ingredients, all packets should be stored in airtight containers and free from damp. Please always use your best judgment when cooking with raw ingredients. Please make sure you are not allergic to any ingredients before use. Anise & Green is not responsible or liable for any reactions that might result from following the recipes. Your health is your responsibility.

You are responsible for ensuring the health and safety of your kitchen, food preparation and storage and for following the instructions provided for your appliances.

4. Anise & Green in no way provides any warranty, express or implied, regarding the content of recipes in this book. The information you read here is believed to be accurate at the time of writing, however changes to information, products and supplies may occur in the future. Anise & Green warmly accepts feedback and suggestions for future editions.

ACKNOWLEDGEMENTS

Thanks to family for your support and encouragement, without which this book would not have been possible.

And thanks to you, the reader, for supporting small steps towards a kinder, more socially and ecologically sustainable way of life.

INDEX

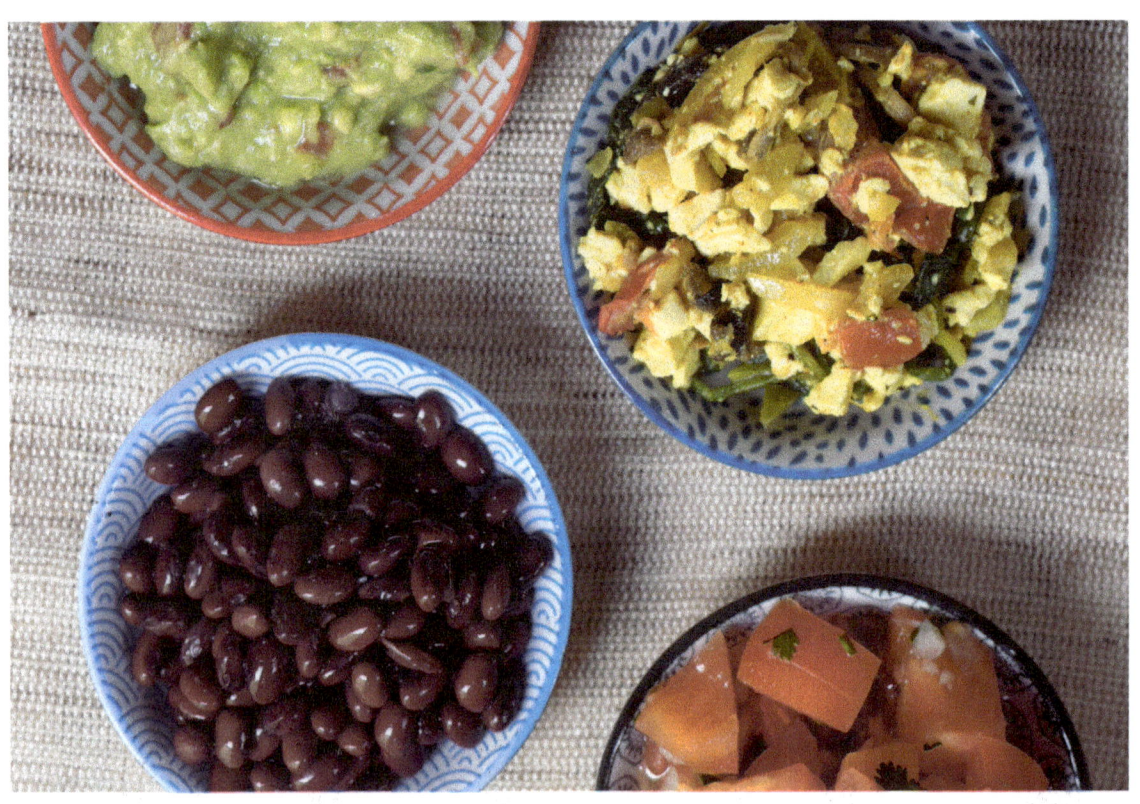

A

almonds 3, 9, 51, 63, 80, 140, 143, 150, 158
amaranth 15, 115
amino acids 2, 14
antioxidants 4, 9, 10, 12, 13
apricots 63

B

barley 3, 26
Barley 15
beans 9, 32
   black beans 39, 56
   butter beans 32
   cannelloni beans 32, 95, 140, 144
   great northern beans 32, 144
   navy beans 32
   pinto beans 32
   white beans 140, 144
beetroot 44
black gram 51
black salt 8, 9, 36, 52, 56, 103, 107, 111, 130
blender 5
blood-sugar 15
blueberries 150
bok choy 22
broccoli 88
buckwheat flour 139

C

calcium 10, 14
calorie 1, 2, 4, 8, 113, 125, 149, 150
cannelloni beans 32
capsicum bell pepper 26, 47, 68, 96, 99
carbohydrates 2, 3, 4, 15
carrots 9, 21, 25, 26, 29, 51, 75, 80, 84, 92, 120, 123, 129
cauliflower 59, 87
cheesy sauce 72
chia seeds 10
   black 136
chickpeas 9, 40
cocoa nibs 10, 143
cocoa powder 10, 139, 143
coconut 10, 147
   coconut cream 67, 76, 147
   coconut flakes 143
   coconut flour 10, 115
      fine 139
   coconut oil 139
   desiccated 150
'complete' protein 3
conversion charts 161
cooking temperature 5, 161
counting calories 1
counting macros 2
couscous
   fine 96
   pearl 116
crumb 36, 92, 115
curry 59, 76

D

daikon radish 119
dates 8, 143, 154
desiccated coconut 10
Desserts 135
   almond flaked rice 140
   choc almond dessert 143
   choc churros 139
   melon coconut dream dessert 147
   raisin & cinnamon semolina 144
   strawberry mousse 136
   dough sticks 35
Dressings 125
   French vinaigrette 126
   lemon caesar dressing 130
   olive mayonnaise dressing 133
   roast carrot dressing 129
Drinks 149
   chai latte 157
   green smoothie 153
   seasonal, coconut & almond oat smoothie (blueberry) 150
   turmeric latte 154

E

ecologically sustainable 7, 8, 10
edamame 120
egg replacement 10
EVOO 12
exercise 4
extra-firm tofu 115

F

FairTrade 10
fats 3
fibre 3
flaked rice 140
flaxseed 10, 139, 150
freekeh 15, 83
fruit 3, 7, 8, 149, 150, 153

G

garlic press 5
ginger 5, 7, 26, 154
glycemic index (GI) 9, 15

grains 15
great northern beans 32
greens 3, 95, 116, 119, 149
guacamolé 56

H

hemp humus & dough sticks 35
hemp oil 11
hemp seeds 11, 35
high protein 2
high-protein 1, 10, 17

I

immune-boosting compounds 11
iodine 8
iron 10, 13, 14

K

kecap manis 13
kidney beans 9
kiwi fruit 11, 153
kombu 12

L

leftover food 17, 32, 95, 103
legumes 9
lentils 9, 25, 75
  orange lentils (red lentils, masoor dahl) 25, 71
  urad dahl (split lentils, black gram) 51
lifestyle 4
linseed 10

M

macronutrients 2
Mains 55
  capsicum roasted tofu 68
  cauliflower queso 87
  cheesy herbed peppers 96
  Chinese tofu 91
  colcannon bowl 95
  easy cheesy pasta 72
  freeky risotto 83
  lemon glazed tofu steak 84
  millet pilaf 80
  mushroom penné 60
  no meat shepherd's pie 75
  peanut & sweet potato tofu stack 79
  roast carrot cutlets 92
  sorghum broccoli risotto 88
  spinach risoni 64
  tantalising tortillas 56
  tempeh curry 76
  tempeh medley 63
  tempeh satay 67
  tempeh tomato stacks 71
  teriyaki tofu 100
  tofu Mediterranean scramble 103
  tofu skewers 99
  yellow tofu curry 59
malt extract 11
marinade 15, 36, 68, 80, 91, 92, 99, 100, 115
Marinades 105
  garlic and ginger marinade 107
  lemon marinade 110
  lime & coriander marinade 111
  spiced warm marinade 108
  sweet and sour marinade 109
  tomato & chilly marinade 106
measures 161

cups 161
spoons 161
melon 147
methionine 11, 12
micronutrients 3, 4, 14
millet 80
mirin 11, 29, 100, 119
miso 11, 22, 119
  miso dressing 119
molasses 8, 11
mushrooms 12, 18, 83, 103
  portobello 96
  shiitake 22, 60

N

nori 12
nutritional yeast flakes 12

O

oats 150
olive oil – extra virgin (EVOO) 12
omega-3 2, 10, 14
omega-6 14
orange lentils (red lentils, Masoor dahl) 25, 71
organic 7

P

paprika 47
pasta 4, 72
  penné 60
  risoni
  orzo 64
peanut chutney 79
peanuts 67, 79, 120
pearl barley 26
peas 9, 59, 75, 88

pilaf 80
polenta 36, 71, 92
protein 1, 2, 3, 4, 9, 10, 11, 14, 15
protein powder 4

Q

queso sauce 87
quinoa 75, 119

R

raw 5, 8, 9, 14, 149
recommended daily intake (RDI) 2
rice 3, 4
  red 119
risotto 83, 88

S

Salads 113
  amaranth tofu salad with lemon dressing 115
  campur dipping salad 120
  pearl couscous spinach salad 116
  quinoa and red rice miso salad 119
salt 7, 8
satay 67
sautéing 5
seasonal and regional 7
seasonal fruit 7, 150
seasonal vegetables 59, 88, 95, 103
seasoning 7
seaweed 12, 84
seeds 9
seitan 3
selenium 12
semolina 144
sesame seeds 12, 29, 40, 84, 91, 99, 100, 115, 119
slimming 2
Snacks and dips
  black bean lime & coriander dip 39
  creamy garlic aioli dip 52
  hot green paprika paté 47
  pea & sweetcorn nuggets and garlic aioli 51
  roasted beetroot dip 44
  sorghum popcorn 43
  spicy salsa dip 48
  spinach humus 40
  tofu bites 36
soaking 9
sorghum 15, 43, 88
Soups 17
  carrot & carroway soup 21
  dahl soup 25
  miso & tofu soup 22
  mushroom soup 18
  sweet potato, ginger & barley 26
  sweet potato, pea & miso soup 29
soy 2
soy beans 13, 158
soy chunks 15, 83
soy milk 5, 13, 18, 44, 47, 52, 59, 60, 64, 71, 72, 75, 83, 87, 95, 96, 129, 133, 140, 143, 144, 149, 150, 153, 154, 157, 158
soy milk maker 158
soy sauce 13
spelt flour 35
spice bag 5
spices 7
spinach 13, 40, 63, 64, 80, 103, 116, 153
split lentils 51
stevia 8, 14
strawberries 136
sugar 3, 8, 15
sunflower kernels 13, 158
supplements 4
sweetcorn 51, 59, 80, 96
sweetener 8, 14
sweet potato 9, 21, 26, 29, 75, 79, 92, 95, 120

T

tahini 35, 40
tempeh (tempe) 3, 14, 63, 67, 71, 76
tofu 14, 15
  dried 22
  extra-firm 36, 91, 92, 99
  firm 56, 59, 68, 80, 84, 91, 99, 100, 115
  firm tofu 26, 116
  freezing 105
  fried 26, 120
  marinating 15, 105
  pressing 105
  semi-firm 79, 103, 120
  silken 14, 44, 47, 52, 119, 129, 130, 133, 143
  soft 29, 44, 47, 52, 123, 129, 130, 133, 136, 143, 147
tomatoes 48, 68, 75, 99, 106, 116, 119
tomato sauce 71
tortillas 56
turmeric 149, 154
TVP - textured vegetable protein 15, 51, 75

V

vanilla essence 15, 139, 147, 154, 158
vegetables 3, 7, 9, 149
  seasonal 59, 88, 95, 103
vitamin A 9, 13
vitamin D 12, 14
vitamin E 9, 11, 13
vitamins 3, 8, 11, 12, 13, 14

W

wakame 12
walnuts 3, 95
weight loss 1
weights and measures 5, 161
whole grains 4, 15
  amaranth 115
  freekeh 83
  millet 80
  sorghum 43

Z

zucchini 51, 59, 84

ANISE & GREEN: THE HIGH-PROTEIN PLANT-BASED COOKBOOK

www.ingramcontent.com/pod-product-compliance
Lightning Source LLC
Chambersburg PA
CBHW061806290426
44109CB00031B/2947